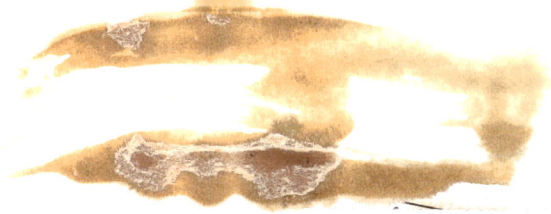

understanding
PATHOLOGY

understanding
PATHOLOGY

*From Disease Mechanisms
to Clinical Practice*

Jeremy R. Jass

*Department of Pathology
Graduate School of Medicine
University of Queensland
Herston, Australia*

harwood academic publishers

Australia • Canada • China • France • Germany • India • Japan • Luxembourg
Malaysia • The Netherlands • Russia • Singapore • Switzerland

Copyright © 1999 OPA (Overseas Publishers Association) N.V. Published by license under the Harwood Academic Publishers imprint, part of The Gordon and Breach Publishing Group.

Amsteldijk 166
1st Floor
1079 LH Amsterdam
The Netherlands

British Library Cataloguing in Publication Data

Jass, Jeremy R.
    Understanding pathology : from disease mechanisms to
    clinical practice
    1. Histology, Pathological
    I. Title
    6.11′.01815

ISBN 90-5702-468-3

CONTENTS

PART I

ANATOMICAL PATHOLOGY: AN EVOLVING AND INTEGRATING DISCIPLINE

PART II

INJURY, INFLAMMATION AND IMMUNITY

PART III

BLOOD, TUBES, FLUIDS AND FLOW

PART IV

NEOPLASIA

PART V

MESSENGERS, METABOLISM, MULTISYSTEM AND MECHANICAL DISEASE

PREFACE

In an era of rapid change and information overload, the student of medicine or health science may become bewildered and disillusioned. The intention of this book is to ground such students by showing how the discipline of pathology fits into society and interfaces with science and medicine. In the new era of integration, the traditional discipline based approach to medical education is over. Yet each discipline must wish to preserve and transmit an essential kernel of understanding. This book represents a personal account of what must remain of the discipline of pathology when the excess is peeled away.

The text focuses on anatomical pathology (histopathology) and the early chapters cover the practice of laboratory medicine in the clinical setting. It is unusual for traditional textbooks of pathology to mention let alone commence with practice. Yet modern pathology and diagnostic laboratory medicine are synonymous. The study and teaching of disease mechanisms is no longer the exclusive province of the pathologist, but has become generalised into the biomedical arena. Academic boundaries have shifted faster than textbooks.

The remainder of the book is structured according to the major disease categories and provides explanations of the underlying mechanisms. Emphasis is placed on the reactions of cells and tissues to initiating stimuli that may be either genetic or environmental in origin. Important ideas and principles are stressed. These are unfolded in historical context to bring meaning, life and movement into what may otherwise be perceived as a dry and static body of knowledge. The style is deliberately discursive rather than didactic.

Basic information relating to histology, embryology, immunity, molecular biology and genetics is introduced at strategic points. This is in recognition of the fact that problem based learners may struggle with concepts for the want of fundamental prerequisite knowledge.

Systemic pathology has been omitted as it is well covered in standard student texts. However, a thorough understanding of an individual disease requires integration across all relevant disciplines. System based specialist texts are a useful source of up to date information that brings both depth and clinical integration to common disorders. Students should be able to pass directly from this text to advanced specialist texts.

ACKNOWLEDGEMENTS

I have attempted to cover a wide field in the interests of integration and uniformity. Neverthe-less, students of medicine and health science are expected to digest an even wider field of study. Each chapter has been read and criticised by at least one colleague, but I take full responsibility for errors of fact, omission or emphasis. I particularly thank Bryan Campbell, Ken Donald, Gordon Campbell, Clive Harper and most especially my wife Johanna for their invaluable suggestions. I also thank Clay Winterford for converting my crude prototypes into such simple but clear and instructive illustrations and Brenda Mason for her secretarial support.

INTRODUCTION

Let us know our reach

Blaise Pascal

This is a book about disease—its nature, classification and the principles underlying tissue diagnosis. The aim is to bring the reader to a clear and comprehensive understanding of disease. The presentation reflects the experience of disease as encountered in the practice of anatomical pathology (histopathology) rather than other areas of pathology, and encompasses over two thousand years of observation, inquiry and investigation coming together as a coherent system in the twentieth century. Pathology is conceived as an evolving and integrating discipline, interfacing with society, science and medicine (Fig. 1).

This is a short text, but quite unlike a series of 'lecture notes'. The shortness is not achieved by leaving out careful explanations but by the deliberate avoidance of repetition, summaries, theoretical detail and information on specific diseases (which should be sought in larger or reference texts). It is usual for nature to reuse a successful invention over and over again rather than reinvent the wheel. Similarly, the same mechanisms reappear in diseases of different types. Details are therefore provided at one appropriate juncture. Only a brief mention of the same mechanism will be found elsewhere (with a cross-reference to the main account). For this reason, an integrated overview will be best achieved by reading the entire book.

It is in the interest of the patient that health professionals liaise in an effective way with the anatomical pathologist. Consequently the book opens with a description of what the anatomical pathologist does and why (Part I). Strangely, this is a topic that is rarely taught at undergraduate or postgraduate levels (even within the discipline of pathology itself). This account is forward looking and one that is mindful of the radical process of restructuring which is affecting the health profession internationally. The modern anatomical pathologist must provide a service that is clinically relevant, standardised and monitored by programs of quality assurance. The practice of medicine is increasingly evidence and team based. The method of teaching pathology must reflect these changes. This will ensure that the contribution of the anatomical pathologist to patient management is well understood and fully actualised.

The doctor of the future needs to acquire more than a large body of knowledge. Anatomical pathology lends itself to the growth of understanding (the ability to synthesise, integrate

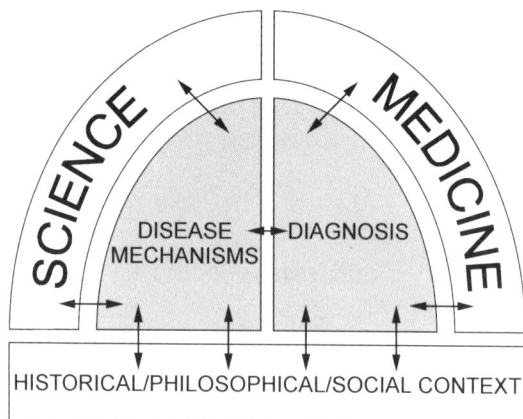

Figure 1 The text focuses on disease mechanisms (general pathology) and the principles of tissue diagnosis (laboratory medicine). There is no system-by-system account of disease processes (systemic pathology). Pathology is 'supported' by its historical, philosophical and social context. Pathology also serves to 'unite' basic sciences with clinical medicine. The text attempts to demonstrate the cohesive and integrating role of pathology and to emphasise that the discipline is more than a 'clinical support service'. It is as an integrated discipline that pathology is best able to serve the needs of both the individual patient and society.

and apply knowledge in an effective manner), the development of skills relating to observation, description and communication, and the acquisition of appropriate attitudes towards disease and its management. This text addresses each of these matters.

Diseases have a cause (aetiology) and show a stepwise process of evolution (pathogenesis). In an ideal world it would be possible to classify a disease by its cause. This ideal cannot be achieved, not only because the initiating cause may not be known but because virtually all diseases are multifactorial. For this reason, it is more realistic to group diseases according to the major underlying pathogenetic process (Table 1). This is the system adopted in Parts II–V of this book. Most important are the inflammatory, cardiovascular and neoplastic disorders and these have been covered in the greatest detail.

The checklist in Table 1 is invaluable. In problem-based learning (PBL) a 'trigger' or piece of clinical information can be matched to one or more of the major disease categories. Two directions may be followed from this point: (1) an exploration of the underlying basic mechanisms, and (2) the development of a list of specific differential diagnoses. An understanding of the mechanisms that explain the responses of cells and tissues to environmental and genetic stimuli is an early priority. Subsequently the emphasis of group learning will shift towards the generation of a broad list of differential diagnoses. The measured release of additional data (clinical and laboratory) will allow the possibilities to be narrowed until there is a final diagnosis that can be fully worked up (Table 2). Mastery of treatment and overall management of a disease is a later goal. However, the achievement of an appropriate diagnosis (or at least a working diagnosis) is a necessary part of management which should never be taken for granted. The ability to reach a diagnosis that is based upon a sound understanding of disease mechanisms has been the key to the success of Western medicine.

Table 1 The twelve categories of disease

1. Inflammatory
2. Cardiovascular
3. Neoplastic
4. Genetic (hereditary)
5. Developmental
6. Endocrine
7. Nutritional
8. Autoimmune
9. Iatrogenic (caused by medical treatment)
10. Mechanical
11. End stage
12. Idiopathic/cryptogenic (cause unknown)

Note: Some diseases fall into two or more categories. Diabetes could be regarded as being genetic, endocrine, nutritional and autoimmune. Diseases may also be classified into those present at birth (congenital) and those acquired later in life. Congenital diseases may be inflammatory (infective), genetic, developmental or mechanical. Genetic disease may not manifest till later in life.

Table 2 The twelve disease descriptors

1. Aetiology (cause)
2. Pathogenesis (mechanisms underlying the evolution of the disease process)
3. Changes at the macroscopic (naked eye) level
4. Changes at the microscopic level
5. Epidemiology (distribution by age, gender, geography, race)
6. Functional effects and clinical features (symptoms and signs)
7. Course or natural history including prognosis
8. Complications
9. Special laboratory investigations for diagnosis, prognosis and monitoring
10. Radiology (diagnostic and monitoring)
11. Preventive strategies
12. Treatment (medical, surgical, palliative, other)

A final diagnosis is sometimes never reached, either because it is undesirable (e.g. in a frail patient), or impossible because of our ignorance of disease. Regrettably, a diagnosis is sometimes missed or made when it is too late to effect a cure. The rare and difficult diagnosis requires a combination of astuteness, firm resolve, a willingness to delve into the literature and a team approach to management which includes the pathologist.

A long journey begins with a desire to reach the destination and proceeds via adequate preparation. This book provides a glimpse of the destination and a few basic provisions. The hero of an epic journey may be faced with a series of deceptively simple riddles. The reader is invited to reflect on the question presented at the beginning of each chapter. The text may not always provide a complete answer, but will hopefully encourage further inquiry.

— PART I —

ANATOMICAL PATHOLOGY

An Evolving and Integrating Discipline

THE ORIGIN AND NATURE
OF PATHOLOGY

*Knowledge of the past and of the places of the earth
is the nourishment of the mind of man*

Leonardo da Vinci

What is the use of history?

The word pathology, derived from the Greek roots *pathos* (suffering) and *logos* (word), means the study of disease. Pathology has therefore been a subject of great and widespread interest throughout history, though the professional pathologist has existed for little more than a century and a half. This may seem surprising, since pathologists are closely linked with human dissection which has been carried out for many centuries.

GRAECO-ROMAN PERIOD

The natural philosophers of ancient Greece carried out human dissection and possibly human vivisection in Alexandria. However, their interest was more in philosophy than medicine, seeking the answer to the command of the Delphic oracle: 'Know thyself'. In Roman times, the body was considered sacrosanct and human dissection was neither permitted nor carried out (despite the opportunities afforded by the mutilated remains of gladiatorial combat). Galen (c.130–201) was born in Pergamum in Asia Minor, studied medicine in Alexandria and practised in Rome, where he became the greatest physician of the age. He wrote of the internal structure of the human body as though he had undertaken dissection himself. However, his words were based on the instruction he had received from his teachers in Alexandria and his personal dissections of animals such as pigs and monkeys. Nevertheless his writings were to become enshrined as the absolute truth on human anatomy until the intervention of Vesalius in the sixteenth century. Galen's views on the cause of disease were the same as those of the Greeks, a holistic belief based on the imbalance of the four humours: yellow bile, black bile, blood and phlegm (Nutton, 1993). Variants of this belief persisted through to the nineteenth century (Maulitz, 1993).

THE MIDDLE AGES

Human dissection began again in the late Middle Ages at the University of Bologna. Canon law permitted the careful external examination of corpses to determine whether inflicted wounds were likely to be the cause of death. During the papacy of Innocent III (1198–1216), it was decreed that a cadaver should be examined by two surgeons and a physician to establish if an earlier blow (inflicted by a bishop during mass) was responsible for the victim's death (Crawford, 1993). By the end of the thirteenth century human dissection for legal reasons was accepted practice in Bologna and this paved the way for the anatomists. The first to undertake human dissection for the purposes of anatomical demonstration was Mondino de Luzzi (c.1275–1326), publishing his *Anathomia* in 1316. He was assisted by two women, Allesandra Gillani and Anna Morandi Mahzolini, who prepared wax models and casts of human organs as educational aids. Within the University of Bologna considerable authority was invested in the students themselves. Should medical students succeed in 'obtaining' a body they were entitled to insist that it be dissected there and then. The history of grave-robbing can be traced back to the Middle Ages.

Dissection was eventually formalised into an annual ritual in Bologna, Padua and other universities in Italy and subsequently other European centres (French, 1993). This took place in winter and continued over a period of three days. The order of the dissection was always the same — abdomen, thorax, cranium and limbs — although Mondino de Luzzi did not extend his own dissections to the limbs. The aim was to demonstrate anatomy, specifically a version of Galen's account as developed by Mondino de Luzzi. The Professor of Anatomy did not undertake the dissection, but oversaw the procedure, demonstrating the findings with reference to Mondino's *Anathomia*. The Professor of Anatomy provided the major intellectual force to the study of medicine during the Middle Ages and Renaissance.

The contribution of the Arab world to the advance of medicine in the second half of the first millennium was considerable. Although the Arabs did not perform human dissection, they translated Galen's writings (in Greek) to Arabic. The original Greek sources were subsequently lost and the Latin versions of Galen used during the Middle Ages were based on translations from the Arabic. Despite the fact that Galen did not see a human dissection, his observations based on animal dissections and translated from Greek through Arabic to Latin were regarded as more reliable than the direct evidence obtained through human dissection. When there was a discrepancy, the fault lay with the corpse, not the writings of Galen! Perhaps man had degenerated since the time of the Graeco-Roman era!

THE RENAISSANCE

The Renaissance was characterised by an intense interest in the ancient world, and scholars rediscovered the original Greek sources of Galen's work. For a period this gave Galen's observations still greater authority, but it was the Brussels born anatomist Andreas Vesalius (1514–1564) who surmised correctly that Galen had not actually witnessed any human dissections. This realisation caused considerable controversy, because the Galenic writings had effectively been incorporated into the Catholic faith and Vesalius was therefore challenging the Church by believing the evidence of his own eyes. As Professor of Anatomy in Padua, he introduced the novel approach of conducting dissections personally and demonstrating the findings with the aid of an articulated skeleton and detailed life-sized engravings. Yet the underlying motivation of ritualised dissection remained as the exposition of the structural complexity of man's hidden interior, in turn providing a glimpse into the mind of the Creator. This philosophical ideal was regarded as more important than any medical benefit and dissection was not conducted for the purposes of explaining disease. This was also the source of fascination for Leonardo da Vinci (1452–1519) who undertook human dissection and illustration as part of his insatiable pursuit of knowledge. Michelangelo (1475–1564) also dissected, largely to understand the sculptural contours of muscles and bones and so imbue his art with greater realism.

SEVENTEENTH CENTURY

It was not until the seventeenth century that human dissection began to be undertaken to determine the cause of death when the cause was known to be natural and not associated with suspicious circumstances. Pictorial records throughout this century depict the officially sanctioned anatomical dissection, a well-known example being *The Anatomy Lesson* by Rembrandt (1606–1669). These ritualised annual occasions were often conducted as a public spectacle fuelled by prurient interest at the prospect of seeing a corpse, not uncommonly that of a notorious criminal, gutted and dismembered as though this were a final and well-deserved punishment. This would have the effect of increasing the perceived sanctity of the body of non-transgressors and impeding the wider practice of autopsy as a means of comprehending the cause of death. Therefore, it is likely that autopsies undertaken to determine the cause of death were performed on poor or neglected individuals with no next of kin. However, the transition from annual anatomical dissection to autopsy for explaining death marks a major turning point in medical history.

In Rembrandt's painting *The Anatomy Lesson*, Nicholas Tulp (1593–1674) displays the anatomy of the muscles of the left forearm of the body of an executed criminal (Schupbach, 1982). His left hand demonstrates the function of these muscles. Tulp was a religious man and his attitude in this painting is indicated in the following contemporary poem by Barlaeus (1645):

> *Evil men, who did harm when alive, do good after their deaths: Health seeks advantages from Death itself.*
> *Dumb integuments teach. Cuts of flesh, though dead, for that very reason forbid us to die.*
> *Here, while with artful hand he slits the pallid limbs, speaks to us the eloquence of learned Tulp:*
> *'Listener, know thyself! and while you proceed through the parts, believe that, even in the smallest, God lies hid'.*

Tulp was also a physician, but as a demonstrator of anatomy he would have been well able to perform autopsies on his patients. This he did, leaving records of correlations between his diagnoses and diseased or morbid anatomy in *Observationes Medicae* (1641). The word 'autopsy' means seeing for oneself. Although Tulp was one of the first to see and illustrate abnormal anatomy that could offer an explanation for death, he was not unique in this regard in the seventeenth century. Other exponents included Theophile Bonet (1620–89) in France, Thomas Willis (1621–1675), the leading English anatomist of this period, and John Brown (1642–c.1700). John Brown was born in Norwich and practised surgery at St. Thomas's

Hospital in London. He had expertise in the management of tumours and was appointed as surgeon to Charles II and William III. In 1665, he communicated the first description of cirrhosis of the liver to the Royal Society of London. His detailed account was based upon the postmortem examination of a 25-year-old soldier who died of liver failure (Major, 1978c).

THE ENLIGHTENMENT

The two types of dissection, anatomical and pathological, continued side by side into the eighteenth century, but it was anatomical dissection that represented the central pillar of medical knowledge and took pride of place in medical school education. The concept of dissection being the final punishment of the poor and wicked was perpetuated in this century by the English painter William Hogarth (1697–1764) in a series of engravings entitled *The Four Stages of Cruelty*. In engraving 3 Tom Nero is caught murdering his mistress. After his death by hanging, his body is shown in engraving 4 being ceremoniously dissected at the Royal College of Physicians, the somewhat disinterested President taking the role of the traditional anatomist. Nero's heart is greedily consumed by a dog (Burke & Caldwell, 1968).

There were still no professional pathologists in the eighteenth century. Autopsy to determine the cause of death when this was already known to be due to a natural cause remained as a rarely performed option for the interested physician. However the Professor of Anatomy in Padua, Giovanni Battista Morgagni (1682–1771) (working in the same dissection theatre as Vesalius two centuries before), kept meticulous records of his 640 postmortem examinations and towards the end of his career he published his life's work, *De sedibus et causis morborum* (The Seat and Cause of Disease). He recognised the importance of altered anatomy as an indication of the cause of disease and carefully correlated what he observed with the patient's life history. He sagely noted that: 'Those who have dissected or inspected many bodies have at least learned to doubt, when others, who are ignorant of anatomy and do not take the trouble to attend it, are in no doubt at all'. Morgagni's single scientific publication heralded the establishment of the autopsy as a powerful scientific tool.

Another factor which encouraged the development of pathology was the growth of an intellectual movement occurring throughout Europe founded on an 'enlightenment' that encompassed rationalism and anticlericalism. Jeremy Bentham (1748–1832), the English legal theorist and reformer and originator of the influential doctrine of utilitarianism, had the final word on the utility of the body as vehicle for teaching. He requested in his will that his skeletal remains be dressed and displayed in the university that he co-founded, University College, London. He made a more practical contribution, however, in the form of the Anatomy Act (1832), passed in the year of his death. Prior to this, the growth of private institutions for the teaching of medicine had resulted in a huge demand for cadavers which could not be met by the relatively small number of executed criminals. The shortfall was made good by the 'resurrectionists' or grave-robbers. The entire enterprise led to riots and the destruction of dissecting rooms by angry mobs (French, 1993). Bentham was opposed to capital punishment, but also perceived the importance of anatomical dissection. The Anatomy Act allowed bodies other than those of executed criminals to be dissected. This included body donation prior to death, which Bentham encouraged through his personal brand of body disposal. In practice the new generation of cadavers consisted of the unclaimed bodies of paupers, and dissection thus became a 'punishment' of the poor as well as the wicked.

NINETEENTH CENTURY

In the late eighteenth and early nineteenth centuries, Parisian physicians including Xavier Bichat (1771–1802) and René Laennec (1781–1826) (inventor of the stethoscope) conducted numerous autopsies on their own patients. Postmortem examination subsequently became more widely practised through the establishment of university chairs of pathology and institutes devoted to the study of pathology. Jean Cruveilhier (1791–1874) was appointed to the first professorship of pathological anatomy in Paris in 1836. He produced an elegantly illustrated atlas of pathological anatomy and is remembered for his accurate illustrations of gastric ulcers. It was not unusual for eminent individuals to be examined postmortem, an early example being Ludwig van Beethoven (1770–1827). In attendance at this occasion was the 23-year-old Karl Rokitansky (1804–1878). After graduating in medicine, Rokitansky specialised in pathology at the Vienna Hospital, becoming Professor of Pathology at the University of Vienna in 1844. Rokitansky devoted all his time to autopsy examinations, claiming to have performed 30,000 by 1866. By this time pathology, spawned from the discipline of anatomy, had replaced the older discipline as the cornerstone of academic medicine. Postmortem examination spread from Europe to America, mainly through the emigration of talented physicians from Germany. The surgeon and reformer of medical education Adam Hammer (1818–1878) settled in St. Louis, Missouri in 1848. In 1876 he commented: 'Obtaining an autopsy in America is attended by great difficulties. How often I have purchased this permission by giving up my fee for professional services! Indeed in certain cases I have had to pay money out of my own pocket to succeed. Before this universal medium even the most subtle misgivings, even the religious ones, soften' (Major, 1978a).

Despite his eminence and unrivalled knowledge of disordered anatomy, Rokitansky still believed that the fundamental cause of disease lay in the imbalance of a humoral or fluid-based factor. It would take a still greater intellect to challenge this doctrine handed down from the Greeks through the writings of Galen. But something new and important was happening. The light microscope, used systematically for the first time by the Netherlandish naturalist Antony van Leeuwenhoek (1632–1723), had been greatly refined and was being applied extensively by the German pathologist Rudolf Virchow (1821–1902). Histopathology (meaning the microscopic examination of diseased tissues) was to evolve from microscopic anatomy via the influence of Virchow, just as the postmortem examination had evolved from anatomical dissection two centuries before.

Virchow was a staunch campaigner for social justice and his outspoken criticisms of the Prussian government led to his dismissal from his post in Berlin. He moved to Würzburg where as professor of pathology and director of the Pathology Institute of Würzburg he developed the concept of 'omnis cellula a cellula' (all cells are derived from cells). Virchow advanced the notion of the cell as the unit of life, that all cells including cancer cells arose from pre-existing cells, and that disease could be understood properly only by studying it at the tissue or microscopic level. His publication *Cellular Pathology* (1858) described the microscopic features of cancer and opened the possibility of diagnosing cancer with the aid of the microscope. Virchow believed that his 'sick cell' theory applied to all disease and did not accept the view that some diseases could be caused by infection with microbes originating in the environment. Nevertheless, his contribution was seminal and revolutionary, underpinning the modern era of clinical practice, clinical research and biomedical research in relation to cancer. When the chair of pathology in Berlin became vacant, the faculty of the university petitioned successfully for Virchow's reinstatement. Virchow accepted the post in

1858 on the condition that the government build him a new institute. His fame became so great that the government acceded to his demand (Major, 1978b).

TWENTIETH CENTURY

It took several decades for pathologists to take up diagnostic work at the microscopic level, the autopsy being perceived as the only legitimate pursuit. In Europe and America, surgeons began to appreciate the value of an accurate diagnosis before undertaking a potentially dangerous procedure and learned the technique of microscopic examination of biopsies. This, however, did not become widespread practice until well into the twentieth century. Up until 1910 surgeons at the Glasgow Royal Infirmary did not value preoperative biopsy, being content for pathologists to confirm or correct the diagnosis of cancer following mastectomy (Jacyna, 1988). Surgeons also began to appreciate the importance of examining operative specimens as a means of evaluating the procedure. By the early twentieth century, laboratory examination and diagnosis of tissue samples was largely the province of the pathologist and has remained so to this day. Nonetheless, anatomical pathology or histopathology has continued to play a prominent role in surgical training and research and the discipline is still sometimes described as surgical pathology, particularly in America. In Japan, surgeons have maintained the tradition of dissecting their own surgical specimens, a fact which emphasises that anatomical pathology is very much part of the process of patient management and not simply a screening or monitoring service.

SUMMARY

This brief overview of the origins of anatomical pathology or histopathology has shown how the discipline developed from anatomical dissection in the seventeenth century, taking a further two hundred years to mature into a specialty that came to be viewed as the cornerstone of medical practice by the latter half of the nineteenth century. In the last 100 years anatomical pathology has been further strengthened by the development of new technologies that will be addressed in subsequent chapters. Nevertheless, the full potential of the discipline has still not been realised.

REFERENCES

Burke, J. & Caldwell, C. (1968) *Hogarth: The Complete Engravings*. London: Thames & Hudson.

Crawford, C. (1993) Medicine and the law. In *Companion Encyclopedia of the History of Medicine*, volume 2, edited by W.F. Bynum and R. Porter, pp. 1619–40. London and New York: Routledge.

French, R. (1993) The anatomical tradition. In *Companion Encyclopedia of the History of Medicine*, volume 1, edited by W.F. Bynum and R. Porter, pp. 81–101. London and New York: Routledge.

Jacyna, L.S. (1988) The laboratory and the clinic: the impact of pathology on surgical diagnosis in the Glasgow Western Infirmary, 1875–1910. *Bulletin of the History of Medicine,* **62,** 384–406.

Major, R.H. (1978) *Classic Descriptions of Disease* (3rd edn), pp. 424–428(a), 508–510(b), 632–635(c). Springfield, Illinois: Charles C. Thomas.

Maulitz, R.C. (1993) The pathological tradition. In *Companion Encyclopedia of the History of Medicine*, volume 1, edited by W.F. Bynum and R. Porter, pp. 169–191. London and New York: Routledge.

Schupbach, W. (1982) *The Paradox of Rembrandt's 'Anatomy of Dr. Tulp'*. London: Wellcome Institute for the History of Medicine.

2

BECOMING A PATHOLOGIST

Obtain knowledge, and then proceed to practice,
which is born of knowledge

Leonardo da Vinci

Why be a pathologist?

APTITUDE AND TRAINING

The anatomical pathologist must be a quick and natural observer and capable of linking this skill to a careful and rigorous approach to the study of disease. A good visual memory is required and the ability to integrate observations of disease with clinical practice. The conclusions then need to be transmitted promptly and unambiguously.

Before becoming an anatomical pathologist, one has to qualify as a doctor of medicine, complete at least one year as a hospital intern and be registered as a medical practitioner. Many gain further clinical experience before embarking on the five years of postgraduate training that is the usual time that it takes to become an accredited anatomical pathologist. The same period of training is required for the other branches of pathology: chemical pathology, haematology and microbiology. Such a protracted period of training is the same for all countries and indeed is typical for all medical specialties. Many people are unaware that consultants or specialists in pathology are medically qualified. There is also the perception that even if pathologists were once medically qualified, the transition to pathology somehow negates this fact and that pathologists are no longer 'real' doctors. This view is of course based on the notion that pathologists do not see patients (except perhaps after death). This notion is in itself incorrect. It is traditional, for example, for chemical pathologists to have clinics for diabetic patients, for haematologists to look after patients with blood disorders, and for microbiologists to manage patents with infections. Although anatomical pathologists may not necessarily have direct contact with patients, some do so when undertaking procedures such as obtaining fine needle aspiration samples (a convenient and painless way of obtaining diagnostic material from a lump).

The postgraduate training required to become an anatomical pathologist occurs on an apprentice basis within institutes whose facilities have been approved by organisations such as the royal colleges in the regions represented by the old British Empire, state boards in the USA, or universities elsewhere. Universities play an indirect role in all countries insofar as teaching institutes are often university medical schools or hospitals with university affiliations. A high proportion of pathologists have a university position and title. The discipline's professional examination is conducted by royal colleges, state boards or universities and provides an important means of establishing high standards of practice. The examination occurs in parts spread over about five years. The early examinations aim to test the aptitude and potential ability of the candidate. The final examination ensures that the trainee has sufficient experience to work safely, independently and to know the limits of his or her ability.

WHY RENOUNCE DIRECT PATIENT CONTACT?

The doctor–patient relationship is a form of human interaction that has enormous emotional force. This is illustrated abundantly by the medium of television and cinema, in which scenes of medical activity include wards, waiting rooms, consulting rooms, accident and emergency rooms, operating rooms, hospital entrances, and even dreary underground passage ways, but rarely, if ever, laboratories — unless the morgue area could be called a laboratory!

In recognition of the appeal of patient contact, modern medical education is increasingly structured upon the early introduction of clinical scenarios or patient-based teaching. The intention is to foster interest in the underlying basic sciences through the demonstration of their direct clinical relevance. While it is necessary for pathologists to have a thorough and clinically-based medical training, career paths aimed towards the investigative disciplines that underpin diagnosis (e.g. pathology and radiology) may be less apparent in courses that are exclusively patient based (since these disciplines may be perceived merely as support services and not clinical specialties in their own right). Why, after many years of training and anticipation of a direct contribution to patient care should a doctor choose a different path leading to the laboratory?

I am not aware of any study on why doctors become pathologists. Obviously most doctors are unwilling to renounce direct patient contact, which is just as well since pathology is a small specialty. Is it renunciation or is it escape from the chaos and pressure that is the lot of the junior hospital doctor? I was once informed that the existence of the specialty was fortuitous because it provided a career option for doctors with personality disorders! While this might appear somewhat extreme, there is the general perception that pathologists do not enjoy interacting with people. If this were so, becoming a pathologist would be inappropriate; the job provides no escape from personal interaction, albeit with clinicians and laboratory technologists. However, it does allow integration of quiet reflection and study into one's daily work.

With regard to patient contact, there are ethical reasons for severing contact between patient and pathologist. The pathologist generates specific diagnostic information and this has to be addressed within the totality of clinical, personal and social factors pertaining to the patient. It is not logistically possible for the pathologist to have such an overview and for this reason overall charge of the patient's care has to be renounced. The actual situation places the patient under the care of a clinician who is expected to piece together all the relevant information. In this capacity the clinician consults the pathologist for a specialist opinion. The information generated by the pathologist is frequently of very major importance to the patient and is gathered in the context of a profound understanding of the clinical significance of the condition in question.

THE CHALLENGE OF DIAGNOSIS

There are other factors that might influence one's decision to become a pathologist. The junior hospital doctor encounters a different aspect of pathology to that presented in medical school. Pathology has immediate clinical relevance and importance, impacting directly on diagnosis and prognosis, and therefore determining subsequent management. Microscopic study and reporting is conducted in an environment that is relatively calm and serene, contrasting with the relative chaos and unpredictability of clinical work. When a complex or rare disorder presents, it is often the pathologist who unravels the mystery and explains the findings. The pathologist clearly belongs to the line of high priests of medical science that can be traced back to the origins of Western medicine. In light of this, pathology can be perceived not as a fusty backwater, but as the living heart of medical practice. The pathologist provides the filter and point of convergence for a range of perplexing or unusual medical condition that turns up in the institution. Unfortunately, the realisation that a career in anatomical pathology might be intellectually satisfying usually comes too late for those who come to appreciate it.

MEDIA AND THE AUTOPSY

The media presents a distorted view of pathology, focusing on forensic pathology and autopsy examination of persons dying under violent, unnatural or even supernatural circumstances. Forensic pathology and anatomical pathology are separate disciplines, though most forensic pathologists are fully trained anatomical pathologists. Women are well represented in the field of anatomical pathology, but relatively few become forensic pathologists. Hospital autopsies (see below) are performed by anatomical pathologists (Chapter 5).

The requirement to perform autopsies can serve as a potential deterrent to a career in anatomical pathology. The smell and sight of a fellow human being dissected is not pleasant. The fact that this undertaking has been performed in Europe for hundreds of years is explained by the educational requirement in relation to both anatomy and pathology and also by the insatiable quest for knowledge in relation to normal structure and function as well as to disease mechanisms. The insatiable drive has now been satisfied, since knowledge of normal structure and function at the level of the naked eye inspection of internal organs is essentially complete. The modern hospital autopsy is no longer a product of the innate curiosity of the pathologist, but is conducted for educational purposes (as in the past) and also as a means of audit. The role of autopsy is considered in greater detail in Chapter 5.

I have focused more on what an anatomical pathologist does than on the details of the training required because the work of the pathologist is the least known amongst that of all health care professionals and any aspects that are known are generally misunderstood. In the past, when autopsy was the main occupation of the pathologist, there may have been understandable reasons for concealing such activities from the public gaze. Apart from any distaste that might be associated with the dissection and handling of human organs, there would also be concern of arousing moral outrage against a practice that contravened widespread and instinctive beliefs in the sanctity of the human body. This would have been in keeping with the well-established paternalistic stance of the medical profession. Medicine today is becoming less paternalistic but the role of the autopsy has receded.

THE NATURE OF ANATOMICAL PATHOLOGY

Anatomical pathology is based on the use of the microscope to examine wafer thin sections (about half the thickness of a single red blood cell) to achieve a diagnosis on behalf of a living patient. A diagnosis is reached rather in the same way that an art expert distinguishes a genuine Rembrandt from a forgery — by careful examination supported by education and experience. The central importance of the discipline of anatomical pathology rests upon the provision of an accurate diagnosis. Diagnosis is the hub around which all subsequent therapeutic decisions turn. Medicine is often described as a blend of art and science, and as a medical subspecialty pathology might be perceived similarly. However, I would argue that pathology leans much more towards being a science than an art and its practice is characterised by a meticulous and highly organised approach. It is the key to the success of Western medicine, providing the entire paradigm for the classification (see Table 1), understanding and diagnosis of disease, and has no rivals in any alternative system of medicine.

3

LABORATORY PROCEDURES AND MANAGEMENT

Know then thyself, presume not God to scan;
the proper study of mankind is man

Alexander Pope

What steps are involved in preparing a histological slide?

ROUTINE HANDLING OF TISSUE SPECIMENS

From the perspective of an anatomical pathologist it is surprising how little is known, either by the layperson or even the rest of the health profession, about the laboratory investigation of human tissue. Tissues obtained from the living may range from minute biopsies the size of a pinhead to very sizeable specimens including whole organs. The smallest specimens are generally taken to diagnose rather than treat disease. The largest specimens are usually organs or parts of organs containing diseased tissue that is life threatening (e.g. a cancer or necrotic tissue).

Tissues arriving at a laboratory specialising in diagnostic anatomical pathology receive considerable care and attention. The management of a tissue sample begins the instant it is removed from a patient (and before it reaches the laboratory), when it is placed in a physiological solution that bathes the tissue in a concentration of buffered salts similar to that of extracellular fluid, thereby preventing cell lysis.

Fixation

The solution into which tissue samples are placed usually includes formaldehyde. First introduced in 1893 (Bracegirdle, 1993), formaldehyde penetrates tissues rapidly and alters the structure of molecules so that all biological activity is destroyed. In particular, enzymes are denatured. This is important, because dying tissues would normally release their own enzymes and digest themselves, a process called autolysis. Dying tissues are also colonised by bacteria, but these are also destroyed by formaldehyde. Formaldehyde thereby preserves normal cellular structure and acts as a mordant, i.e. it facilitates the subsequent staining of the tissues with dyes. The entire process is called tissue fixation (since it attempts to 'fix' tissue in a lifelike state) and takes a few hours to a day or two, depending on the size of the specimen. Fixation can be speeded up by microwaving the tissue.

Sometimes tissues are teased out onto a suitable flat surface, such as a cover slip, before being placed into the fixation fluid. This applies to biopsies of the delicate lining of the intestine which would otherwise curl up into distorted shapes, making subsequent interpretation difficult or impossible. This delays fixation for a few minutes, but this does not matter.

Generally speaking, the best way of preserving tissue when fixation fluids are not at hand is to refrigerate the tissue at 4 °C without placing it in any fluid. Refrigeration slows down the processes within the cell that destroy tissue once it is removed from the body. Freezing will preserve tissues indefinitely (at –80 °C), but must be instantaneous. In a domestic freezer, normal microscopic structure will be destroyed by ice crystal formation.

As well as immersing the tissue specimen in a container containing formaldehyde in buffered saline, it is necessary to attach a label to the pot with the patient's name and hospital number. Getting the right label on the container is obviously of paramount importance. Pathologists cannot pick up a clerical error when consecutive patients undergo similar types of biopsy procedure and get their names swapped on the containers. Additionally a request form is filled in, again with the patient's name, identification number, name of the clinician responsible for the patient's management, an address to send the final report and clinical details about the patient. The specimen and request form are then placed at a pick-up point for collection and delivery to the appropriate laboratory by a hospital porter. In the reception area of the laboratory the pot and form are given a laboratory number and this number and specimen and patient details are logged into a 'day book'. Specimens and request forms are then taken to a 'cut-up' room where they are handled in batches.

Cutting up

The cut-up room is where the specimens are examined, described and dissected by the anatomical pathologist. (There is always a smell of formaldehyde about the place despite the presence of air venting systems.) The description covers the type of specimen including measurements of normal anatomical structures. The pathological 'lesion' is described in terms of its site and relationship to normal structures as well as its size, shape, colour and consistency. For example, if the lesion is believed to be a cancer, the surgical excision margins are marked with a pigment such as india ink. This is visualised later on microscopic examination as a fine black line following the contour of the surgical margin. This serves as proof that this important landmark has been included in the microscopic preparation and also establishes with certainty whether or not the cancer has been completely removed by the surgeon (Quirke et al., 1986).

Large specimens of hollow organs, such as the gut, are opened with scissors, washed in a sink (a short exposure to tap water is not harmful) and pinned out on a board, together with a tag indicating the patient's name and laboratory number. The board is then turned upside down and floated in a large tank of fixation fluid. Detailed dissection is usually deferred to the following day. Dissection involves the selection of small samples of tissue for microscopic examination. These pieces may amount to only a small fraction of the entire specimen, but they should be representative of the organ as a whole and provide all the diagnostic information that is needed. The samples are placed in plastic cassettes with a snap on lid. There are small perforations in the cassette and lid to allow solutions to percolate around the selected tissue when it is processed further. The patient's laboratory number is pencilled onto the edge of the cassette and is not worn off. The cassettes will remain in formaldehyde solution for a further period of time to ensure that the tissue samples are thoroughly fixed. Care must be taken so that clusters of malignant cells from one specimen are not inadvertently transferred to the following patient's tissue sample. To prevent such potentially misleading 'carry over' all surfaces used in dissection are cleaned meticulously between cases.

Processing and staining

The stage of tissue processing follows. This is achieved by automatic processors that remove all traces of water from the tissue, which is passed progressively through 70%, 90% and then two steps of 100% alcohol, and finally a chemical called xylene. If the tissues have been fixed correctly, they will withstand this harsh treatment. The specimens are then removed from the cassettes and oriented within metal moulds into which warm liquid paraffin wax is poured. The plastic cassette is placed on top of the mould while the wax hardens. It then forms a pedestal for the wax cast containing the specimen after it has been removed from the mould.

Suspended in this way in a wax cast, the specimen can be cut into sections about half the thickness of a red blood cell by a laboratory technologist using a microtome. After emerging from the microtome the sections are floated onto a warm water bath, from which one or more is selected and placed onto a glass slide. The frosted end of the slide is marked with the laboratory number and the slides are placed in an oven to dry.

The next stage involves removing the wax and staining the sections. The slides are loaded into racks and placed in xylene to dissolve the wax. This is followed by 100%, 90% and 70% alcohol and finally back to water, whereby the sections become completely transparent. In order to be studied by microscopic examination, they are dyed with chemicals, usually haematoxylin, which stains nuclei blue (due to the presence of acidic DNA) and eosin which imparts a pink colour to the cytoplasm (H&E sections). The sections are then dehydrated and returned to xylene before being covered with a glass cover slip with the aid of runny and transparent mounting medium that slowly hardens. A senior technologist checks the final quality of the slides and then they are passed to the anatomical pathologist for reporting.

Reporting

If the specimen is small and the diagnosis straightforward, a report can usually be dictated, typed and signed out on the same day (i.e. within 24 hours of the receipt of the specimen). The reporting of large or complicated specimens will take longer and delays of two to three days are justified. There are several explanations for delays, apart from the longer fixation time required for large specimens. The samples selected for microscopic study may turn out to be unrepresentative and this will necessitate the selection of additional tissue. Secondly, the disease may be rare or represent a variant of the usual form and the opinion of additional pathologists, perhaps with specialist knowledge, will be needed to complete the report. It is very common practice amongst pathologists to seek a second opinion. This even occurs amongst acknowledged experts and, because of the ready consignment of glass slides by mail, is an undertaking that knows no boundaries. (One of the earliest examples of the international transportation of human tissues would have been the wax injected preparations illustrating the capillary bed of the kidney sent by the Edinburgh physician John Morgan (1735–1789) to the Paduan Professor of Anatomy Giovanni Battista Morgagni (1682–1771) with the assistance of Venetian merchants (Maulitz, 1993).) Finally, it may not be possible to reach a definite diagnosis without performing one or more special stains.

STAINING TECHNIQUES

The principal aim of staining a tissue section for the purposes of microscopic examination is to transform a transparent and almost invisible structure into one that may be made clearly visible when light is projected through it to reach the eye of an observer via the magnifying optics of a microscope. Although the tissues of the body are coloured to the naked eye (brown liver, yellow fat, red blood), they are transparent and colourless when sectioned finely. Plants are similarly insipid, but at least have thick cell walls that impart a distinct microscopic pattern. The cells of human (and animal) tissues are limited by a delicate membrane that is no more than an aggregation of molecules.

The early attempts at tissue staining were achieved by trial and error using natural dyes that had been available and in use for centuries, if not millennia, for dying fabrics. Leeuwenhoek (1632–1723) applied saffron solution to preparations of muscle fibres. By the end of the nineteenth century, the most popular stain for tissue sections was carmine derived from cochineal (Mayer, 1892). Cochineal is a red dye prepared from the dried female bodies of a scale insect, *Dactylopius coccus*. It was known to the Aztecs, the ancient Romans and apparently in biblical times since the Divinity exhorted Moses to prepare offerings of rams' skins dyed red (Exodus 25:5). Orcein, known originally as French purple, dates from the 1300s (AD) when it was prepared from an extract of lichen (a primitive plant that is part fungus and part alga) that was exposed to air in the presence of ammonia formed in fermented urine (Conn, 1948). Orcein is still used for staining various tissue components, but thankfully is now prepared differently. Haematoxylin is derived from the wood of a tree called *Haematoxylon campechianum*, so named because it originated in the Mexican State of Campeche. Synthetic dyes, for example alcian blue developed by ICI, have also been used to stain cell products.

Contrasting with the empirical approach employing natural and synthetic dyes derived from the textile industry is 'designer' staining utilising predicted biochemical reactions between specific reagents (reactive agents) and substrates (biochemical components within the cell upon which reagents act). This may be likened to the controlled biochemistry within a test tube except that the reaction (described as histochemistry) occurs within a tissue section. The substrates may include all manner of biological molecules, for example enzymes, carbohydrates, hormones and even DNA. Histochemistry permits the visual demonstration of molecules in their normal location by means of coloured reagents. The intensity of the colour reaction may even indicate the amount of cellular substrate, as well as its exact site of production within the cell.

The staining of tissue sections is therefore a mixture of old craft and modern science, the result being the visual display of the secrets of cell structure and function that is indeed as spectacular as a stained glass window. The astute reader may have noticed the inclusion of enzymes in the list of biological molecules that can be 'seen', yet these delicate molecules are generally rendered inactive by the process of fixation and thus should not be detectable through their biological activity. Such denaturing of enzymes can be circumvented by preparing unfixed sections from a frozen block of tissue. These 'frozen sections' lack the preservation of structural detail of sections prepared by the traditional method, and the enzyme activities associated with living tissues can be 'seen' within them. There is an additional method of seeing enzymes or any other cellular component and this leads on to an advance in histotechnology of very considerable importance — the use of the monoclonal antibody.

MONOCLONAL ANTIBODIES

Antibodies are relatively large molecules produced by plasma cells which are modified B lymphocytes. As part of the immune defence system of man and 'higher' animals, antibodies attach themselves to antigens on the surface of invading viruses and bacteria, assisting directly and indirectly in their destruction. The regions of antibodies that recognise an antigen show considerable structural variability (see page 85), which is necessary because antigens are of infinite variety. A single plasma cell, however, produces an antibody with only one structure, and this will be specific for one antigenic structure.

Antibodies can be raised artificially by injecting antigenic material into an animal. To achieve production of a specific antibody of a single type that recognises only a single antigen would require difficult purification that would yield very little antibody. Koehler and Milstein (1975) developed a technique for producing very large amounts of monoclonal antibody and their efforts were rewarded with a Nobel prize. Their technique involved the fusion of primed B lymphocytes (obtained from a mouse that had previously been injected with antigen) with malignant and therefore immortal plasma cells. The resulting hybrid cell engineered in the laboratory contained both the specific instruction as well as the machinery to produce antibody. Furthermore, one could begin with a single cell which would divide and produce identical cells (a hybridoma) all secreting the same monoclonal antibody.

Monoclonal antibodies have many uses and their full potential as therapeutic agents is yet to be realised. When used to stain particular chemical structures in cells, their specific binding is amplified using one or more 'layers' of different antibodies and finally visualised with an antibody that is 'complexed' with a chemical that gives a colour reaction (Fig. 2). This technique is called immunohistochemistry and is undertaken routinely in diagnostic laboratories as well as being a powerful research tool. A particularly important use of the monoclonal antibody is in the classification of cancer (Chapter 22).

FROZEN SECTIONS

A small tissue specimen may be 'blocked' in paraffin wax. The blocks and stained sections prepared from each block will be retained in the laboratory for several decades. The remains of large specimens cannot be stored and are usually cremated after one to two months. Mention has been made of frozen sections for visualising enzymes. Frozen sections can also be prepared, stained with H&E and examined by the pathologist in a few minutes. However, interpretation is compromised by poorer preservation of microscopic detail and frozen material cannot be stored conveniently. Nevertheless, pathologists do examine frozen sections when a rapid diagnosis will clearly be of benefit to the patient. The usual example will be during an operation when the findings of the pathologist will guide the surgeon and directly influence the course of the surgical procedure. This was once a common part of the management of breast cancer. (Nowadays, however, the diagnosis of breast cancer is usually made preoperatively by cytological examination of a fine needle aspirate and the patient participates in the decision regarding mastectomy versus simple removal of the lump.) A practical reason for not performing a frozen section during an operation for breast cancer is that cutting into the cancer during surgery distorts the specimen and makes subsequent interpretation by the pathologist difficult. This may impede informed decision making with respect to any need for further surgery.

LABORATORY MANAGEMENT

Pathologists keep strict records of their work. This includes hard copies of all reports as well as computerised records of these which will provide an index of all patients and all diseases that have been diagnosed. Diseases are coded by both anatomical site and type of disease. Modern computers with relational databases will allow searches to be made for any field of study. For example, one may wish to review all cases of carcinoma of the cervix diagnosed within a particular period in order to investigate the potential usefulness of a monoclonal antibody raised against an antigen such as human papillomavirus or the product of a recently identified cancer gene. In the past, separate patient and disease indices were maintained on card systems containing typed or even handwritten data. This was laborious work, but given the overall supervision of an anatomical pathologist, such record systems were the starting point for valuable clinical research spanning many decades. Indeed they often provided the only means of accessing and integrating clinical and pathological data with reference to both disease and patient.

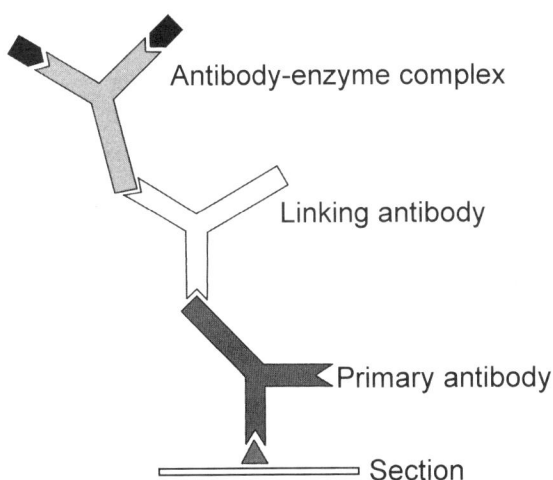

Figure 2 Indirect immunohistochemical technique. The primary monoclonal antibody (mouse) is raised against a tissue antigen. Amplification is achieved with a linking rabbit anti-mouse antibody. The antibody-peroxidase complex represents the third layer of the 'sandwich'. The peroxidase converts diaminobenzidine into a brown visualisable product.

Quality of laboratory practice applies to the stained histological section prepared by the technologist, the diagnostic information provided by the pathologist and the turnaround time. Most laboratories monitor all three as part of quality assurance programs (Zardawi et al., 1998). Laboratories are often subject to official accreditation which takes account of the state of laboratory equipment, adequacy of training of technical staff and the adequacy of health and safety procedures to protect staff from both infection and toxic chemicals. Issues relating to standards of reporting are discussed in subsequent chapters.

REFERENCES

Bracegirdle, B. (1993) The microscopical tradition. In *Companion Encyclopedia of the History of Medicine*, volume 1, edited by W.F. Bynum and R. Porter, pp. 102–119. London and New York: Routledge.

Conn, H.J. (1948) *History of Staining* (2nd edn). Geneva, New York: Biotech Publications.

Koehler, G. & Milstein, C. (1975) Continuous cultures of fused cells secreting antibody of predifined specificity. *Nature,* **256,** 495–497.

Maulitz, R.C. (1993) The pathological tradition. In *Companion Encyclopedia of the History of Medicine*, volume 1, edited by W. F. Bynum and R. Porter, pp. 169–191. London and New York: Routledge.

Mayer, P. (1892) Über das Färben mit Carmin, Cochinille und Hämatein Thonerde. *Mitt Zool Stat Neapel,* **10,** 480–504.

Quirke, P., Dixon, M.F., Durdey, P. & Williams, N.S. (1986) Local recurrence of rectal adenocarcinoma due to inadequate surgical resection. Histopathological study of lateral tumour spread and surgical excision. *Lancet,* **ii,** 996–999.

Zardawi, I.M., Bennett, G., Jain, S. & Brown, M. (1998) Internal quality assurance activities of a surgical pathology department in an Australian teaching hospital. *J Clin Pathol,* **51,** 695–699.

4

THE INTERFACE BETWEEN PATHOLOGY AND CLINICAL MEDICINE

'My wish', cried Don Quixote 'is to serve'

Cervantes

How does communication between clinician and pathologist benefit the patient?

THE CLINICOPATHOLOGICAL AXIS

A certain level of tension characterises the relationship between clinician and pathologist. The source of this tension can be traced to the split of laboratory and clinical (bedside) medicine that occurred in the latter half of the nineteenth century. The split was dramatised in clinicopathological conferences where the clinician would attempt to reach a diagnosis on the basis of the patient's medical history, but the autopsy findings presented by the pathologist would serve as the final word. Furthermore, the laboratory rather than the ward was perceived as forming the epicentre for medical research. In order to succeed in research one had to remove oneself from the care and distraction characterising clinical work. Pathologists who were laboratory based were therefore competent to undertake research and received university recognition long before clinical research was to develop any form of academic coherence (mainly instigated through the medical schools of North America) (Booth, 1993). As full-time academics, pathologists also saw themselves as central to the teaching of medicine. These important and pivotal roles contributed to an exclusiveness that underpinned the establishment of large and powerful departments of pathology. Today much of this exclusiveness has evaporated as many of the traditional activities of the pathologist have dissipated. In a sense the discipline became too large and important for its message to be barricaded within a single framework.

COMMUNICATION

The principal residue of the once formidable discipline of pathology is now preserved in the area of diagnostic service. This involves the clinician requesting a laboratory investigation and the pathologist carrying it out. Much of this happens in a rather mechanical way and can best be illustrated with respect to surgery and the management of cancer. For example, after about an hour of operating, part of an organ is routinely submitted to the anatomical pathologist. The pathologist does not specifically ask for the specimen to be sent and may be unaware of its existence until it is delivered into his/her care. The specimen is accompanied by a request form containing information about the patient's identity and clinical history. Often this is completed by a junior doctor or a nurse. The clinical information may be detailed but sometimes no information is provided at all. Useless or even incorrect information may be supplied and important and/or relevant information may be omitted or be indecipherable. The variable nature of the information transfer is indicative of suboptimal systems of communication. Since clinical information is needed by the pathologist in order to generate a report that is both correct and meaningful, it is necessary for the pathologist to explain its purpose to the clinician. Things are more likely to happen and happen well if they have a purpose that is understood. Surprisingly, there is very little, if any, opportunity to explain such practical and mundane matters to medical students or junior hospital doctors. Completing forms is not a popular activity and is unlikely to arouse sufficient interest to merit space in an increasingly crowded medical school curriculum. Yet neglecting this topic may have dire medical and legal consequences.

In order to interpret a surgical specimen correctly the pathologist must be able to 'see' the patient around it. The specimen needs to be understood in anatomical terms as a three-dimensional object, the surgical margins of which were once joined seamlessly to the patient. In the case of a cancer, the malignant growth will radiate out in all directions and may even reach the limits of the surgical specimen. Any points of surgical transection of cancer will previously have been in contact with tissues remaining in the patient. These tissues will unfortunately contain residual cancer that will continue to grow, cause symptoms and eventually may lead to the patient's death. By knowing the precise location of any residual cancer, the clinician may be able to target further treatment to this area, either in the form of additional surgery or radiotherapy. This serves to illustrate the practical importance of close liaison between clinician and anatomical pathologist.

Communication between the surgeon and the pathologist can be assisted by the actual attendance of the pathologist within the operating theatre. This sometimes occurs but is not feasible as a routine practice because of the relatively smaller number of pathologists in comparison with that of surgeons. An alternative approach is for the surgeon to dissect the specimen following its removal from the patient. As alluded to in Chapter 1, this is usual practice in Japan. However the dissection may take longer than the operation itself and the pathologist is not the same as the person undertaking the dissection. This approach simply means that the continuity of care is broken at a step far removed from the patient and the clinical input by the pathologist is compromised. The most workable solution is for the specimen to be sent to the pathologist in the condition it is in immediately following its removal from the patient. It can be usefully accompanied by a drawing indicating any areas of concern. The surgeon can also mark important points on the specimen with knots of suture material cut at different lengths to facilitate recognition. If the pathologist is still unsure about orientation, an attending surgeon can provide assistance in consultation over the intact specimen in the laboratory.

Sometimes surgeons slice or cut open the specimen themselves to see the area of disease. This is generally undesirable unless the findings might actually alter the course of the surgery in a way that would benefit the patient. Interference with the specimen inevitably produces confusing distortion of the anatomy, making it difficult or impossible for the pathologist to achieve a three-dimensional reconstruction of the sample and understand its relationship to the patient.

There are two major steps in the clinical management of the patient with cancer (the disease that is central to the work of the anatomical pathologist) in which the anatomical pathologist is closely involved and communicates diagnostic information. The first concerns the establishment of the diagnosis of cancer. This is a crucial stage because correct treatment depends absolutely on the diagnosis achieved through the histological examination of a sample of tumour tissue. (The methods of achieving a tissue diagnosis of cancer are described in Chapters 21 and 22.) Tissue samples are obtained by a relatively non-invasive technique such as fine needle aspiration or by means of forceps or scalpel under direct vision. The second step is the examination of the definitive specimen of cancer following the hopefully successful attempt by the surgeon to remove the tumour in its entirety and so cure the patient.

The chapters on cancer forming Part IV of this book encompass the handling of surgical specimens by the pathologist and show how information is generated for the production of a written report that is transmitted to the clinician. The final report contains: (1) patient details (name, date of birth, date of procedure, location — ward or outpatient), (2) name of clinician, (3) clinical details, (4) macroscopic description, (5) microscopic description and (6) final diagnosis. There may also be interpretative comments and/or references to relevant literature in difficult or unusual cases. The report may be accompanied by photographs of the specimen (usually in the form of 35 mm colour slides). However the generation and submission of such a report is not sufficient on its own to ensure optimum standards of patient care. The missing element is the clinicopathological meeting.

CLINICOPATHOLOGICAL MEETING

The two major steps in the pathological management of cancer are reflected in two types of clinicopathological meeting. The first meeting will address the diagnosis of cancer and the second will discuss the major surgical procedure including the expected outcome for the patient. Surgeons are usually interested more in the second type of meeting because the definitive surgical specimen can be reviewed and contemplated as a postscript to the operation. The first type of meeting is generally of greater interest to the pathologist because of the fundamental need for establishing a diagnosis of cancer that is not only correct but extracts all information that may be usefully gained from the exercise, thereby ensuring that decision making on behalf of the patient is optimised.

The microscopic examination of a tissue specimen is the principal procedure for achieving a diagnosis of cancer, but is not an exercise that can be conducted in isolation. The pathologist also requires clinical information regarding the age, sex and race of the patient and the precise site of the tumour. The smaller the biopsy, the greater the need for this additional information if error is to be avoided. The X-ray appearances of some tumours (e.g. bone cancers) may form a crucial component of the diagnostic process. Laboratory results in relation to blood tests may provide essential diagnostic evidence and haematological input may be mandatory for cancers of blood (leukaemia) or lymph nodes (lymphoma). Genetic and molecular biological findings may also be pivotal, adding information that may refine the diagnosis and influence treatment.

It is evident that the correct diagnosis of cancer is very much a team effort. It is now common practice for oncologists, radiotherapists and radiologists to join clinical meetings that focus on cancer management. The job of the pathologist is not merely to study microscopic appearances but to integrate the appearances of structural disorder with the totality of available clinical information. Some clinicians believe that information should be concealed from the pathologist to prevent bias or preconception from influencing the diagnosis. This is dangerous practice giving rise to avoidable errors, and ignores the fact that pathologists are medically qualified and trained to integrate laboratory and clinical information. As in the case of a judge, the pathologist is more likely to reach a correct diagnosis only after all the evidence has been assembled.

THE REFERRED PATIENT

In most cases, diagnosis and treatment is simple and straightforward and there are no problems. However, the initial investigation of a patient with a suspected cancer may occur in centres without special diagnostic expertise. The establishment of the correct and fully detailed diagnosis is an absolute prerequisite for informed decision making in relation to the administration of treatment as difficulties can arise when the cancer is a rare form, has presented at an advanced stage, has occurred in a site where the results of treatment are especially influenced by the level of surgical expertise or where its treatment calls for a team approach.

When the treatment of cancer fails in non-specialist centres it is often not possible to turn the clock back and correct the problem. Alternatively, surgery may be optimal (or considered so), but the postoperative pathological findings may indicate the need for additional treatment in the form of chemotherapy or radiotherapy. If such patients are referred to specialist cancer centres for further management it is customary and good practice for the anatomical pathologist in the cancer centre to review all the earlier pathological material and issue a supplementary report. Such a review rarely leads to revision of the underlying diagnosis, but may result in the detection of microscopic features of diagnostic importance that were not noted earlier (see Chapters 21 and 22).

The main difficulty, however, will relate to reconstruction and understanding of the surgical specimen, specifically the extent of spread and the possible location of the cancer at one or more surgical excision margins. In other words it may not be possible to establish in retrospect if the cancer was removed in its entirety or not. Furthermore the attempt to do so may often consume more time than that required for correct handling in the first place. If the examination was not undertaken properly and in accord with standardised procedures on the first occasion, there is usually no possibility of retrieving the necessary information. The informed planning of further treatment will be seriously compromised.

The situation in which therapeutic decisions have to be made in the absence of appropriate pathological information is a relatively new one. It reflects the increasing availability of new forms of cancer treatment and the growing realisation of the importance of evidence in decision making. The problem is not widely acknowledged and the magnitude of its significance for the patient has not been estimated. Pathologists working in countries that contain large and relatively unpopulated regions served by non-specialist medical centres will be more familiar with the difficulties engendered by professional isolation and poor communication. The current vogue for decentralising health care is exposing weaknesses resulting directly from the break up of informed and integrated teamwork that is so necessary for the proper management of serious and complex medical disorders of which cancer is probably the best example.

One solution for the preceding dilemma is to institute rigorous accreditation of centres engaged in the diagnosis and treatment of cancer (or suspected cancer) that take account of the outcome survival and quality of life of patients treated for the various types of cancer. Since outcome is heavily influenced by the type, grade and extent of spread of the cancer, it is clear that the recording of these parameters by the pathologist must be both standardised and meticulous.

TELEPATHOLOGY

Telemedicine is the transfer of image and sound through computer networks and telepathology is a branch of telemedicine (Dervan & Wootton, 1998). Telemedicine may involve the transfer of static images or real-time dynamic interaction. Telepathology allows the pathologist to achieve remote control use of a distant microscope and this has been used to provide a diagnostic service in relatively sparsely populated countries such as Norway (Nordrum & Eide, 1995). Diagnostic use may be limited to the transfer of selected static images via the Internet to pathologists with special diagnostic expertise (Eusebi et al., 1997). Telepathology has been used less widely than teleradiology, presumably because clinicians like to view and interpret radiological images for themselves (whereas pathological images are left to the pathologist). Nevertheless, telepathology is likely to assume increasing importance in distance learning as well as diagnosis.

REFERENCES

Booth, C.C. (1993) Clinical research. In *Companion Encyclopedia of the History of Medicine*, volume 1, edited by W.F. Bynum and R. Porter, pp. 205–229. London and New York: Routledge.

Dervan, P.A. & Wootton, R. (1998) Diagnostic telepathology. *Histopathology*; **32**, 195–198.

Eusebi, V., Foschini, L., Erde, S. & Rosai, J. (1997) Transcontinental consults in surgical pathology via the Internet. *Human Pathol*, **28**, 13–16.

Nordrum, I. & Eide, T.J. (1995) Remote frozen section service in Norway. *Arch Anat Cytol Pathol*, **43**, 253–256.

5

THE ROLE OF AUTOPSY

Courage is demanded of us to have strength for the strange,
singular and most inexplicable events we may encounter

Rainer Maria Rilke

What is the value of autopsy examination?

ESTABLISHMENT OF AUTOPSY

Human dissection undertaken to explain the cause of a natural death as opposed to a death caused by inflicted injury has a history of nearly four centuries, spanning the ages of enlightenment, reason and the romantic and modern eras. As mentioned in Chapter 1, before the seventeenth century, the main practical use of anatomical dissection was to assist in the training of surgeons and investigate a number of violent deaths. However, these aims were eclipsed by the higher desire to know and appreciate the mind of the Creator through the formal demonstration of man's internal organs. This was clearly a factor in the dissection by Tulp, as described in Chapter 1, but Tulp was also interested in explaining disease through the elucidation of abnormal anatomy. Dissection had a dual role for Tulp: the display of the Creator's work and the corruption of this work through disease. The seventeenth century also saw the expression of a more wide ranging duality of spirit and body through the philosophical writings of René Descartes (1596–1650) and represents a pivotal point between the old God-centred world and the new materialism. By the eighteenth century God and pathological anatomy had parted company, with the full intellectual force of the latter being finally realised in the nineteenth century through the professionalisation of the discipline and the establishment of institutes of pathology and university chairs of pathology across Europe and America.

CLINICOPATHOLOGICAL CORRELATION

In the nineteenth century, the centrepiece of pathological anatomy was the autopsy. Sir William Osler (1849–1919), perhaps the greatest physician of his period, stated: 'To investigate the cause of death, to examine carefully the condition of the organs after such changes have gone on in them to render existence impossible, and to apply such knowledge to the prevention of and treatment of disease is one of the highest objectives of the physician'. The correlation of autopsy findings with the patient's medical history became the quintessential exercise in medical intellectual gymnastics, and was formalised as the clinico-pathological correlation (CPC) through the drive and energy of notable teachers of medicine at Harvard including W. B. Cannon (1871–1945) and Richard Cabot (1868–1939), the latter instigating the publication and dissemination of CPCs as the *Case records of the Massachusetts General Hospital* (Maulitz, 1993).

The CPC procedure involved the disclosure of a clinical record to a guest physician who was expected to exercise his or her critical prowess by arriving at the correct diagnosis (or at least a sensible list of differential diagnoses in decreasing order of likelihood). The reputation of the physician would then be further enhanced if the pathologist provided and demonstrated proof of the suggested diagnosis in terms of diseased anatomy. Despite all the erudition and wisdom displayed by the physician, the pathologist always had the final word in confirming or refuting the diagnosis with the unanswerable and dramatic demonstration of the morbid anatomy. The lasting effect of this process to this day has been to cement the view of the pathologist as the final arbiter of diagnostic accuracy. The effect at the time was to magnify the standing of pathology, but also to place pathology and medicine into distinct compartments, with pathology being removed from the living patient. The singular importance of the autopsy also obscured and impeded the development of more relevant activities, such as the diagnosis of disease before death.

Basking in self-importance, pathologists were slow to pick up and run with the newer offshoots of their own discipline, instead allowing surgeons to develop the art of microscopic diagnosis of tissue specimens removed from the living. However, the perceived self-importance was actually rather limited, pathologists being appreciated mainly by clinical colleagues within the ivory tower environments of the leading medical establishments. Autopsy was not a subject to arouse the interest and support of the wider community. The offshoot of surgical pathology was ultimately incorporated into the business of the anatomical pathologist, but even this most practical activity was (and still is) largely concealed from the public gaze.

INVISIBLE CAUSES OF DEATH

The mechanisms underlying disease and death are not necessarily explained exclusively on the basis of abnormal structure, even when anatomical investigation is supported by the most sophisticated microscopic techniques. More fundamental are the abnormalities relating to biological molecules and their functional orchestration at the level of the cell. Many such biochemical disturbances are revealed in the composition of blood and other body fluids which can be collected and analysed with relative ease. Such clinical biochemistry (or chemical pathology) offers a rapid and powerful approach to diagnosis that complements and in some cases may even replace tissue diagnosis.

MODERN IMAGING

Radiology has contributed an alternative, non-invasive approach to diagnosis that has been strengthened in recent years by the introduction of ultrasound imaging, computerised axial tomography (CAT) and magnetic resonance imaging (MRI), all of which continue to be developed and refined. These techniques generate startlingly clear, detailed and lifelike images of internal organs, both normal and diseased. The organs may even be observed through time, giving an indication of their functional activity. Compared with these newer anatomical modalities that can be applied to the living, autopsy seems crude and outmoded instrument. Yet tissue examination remains as a diagnostic gold standard for many diseases, notably cancer. Furthermore, modern technology has increased the diagnostic potential of anatomical pathology by allowing virtually any organ of the body to be biopsied in life. Indeed, the imaging techniques do not merely stand on their own, but allow guided biopsy instruments to be targeted upon tiny internal lesions that would otherwise be accessible only through surgical intervention.

AUTOPSY AND AUDIT

Notwithstanding the range of diagnostic tools that are now available to the modern clinician, autopsy remains an important forensic procedure, applying to those varied situations in which death has not occurred through natural causes or with the knowledge of an attending medical practitioner. Clinicians may still request a postmortem examination for non-legal purposes when a patient's terminal illness was particularly complex or unusual in some way. Alternatively, the patient may have been too ill to endure extensive investigation in the days or weeks preceding death. Clinicians rarely attend these autopsy demonstrations and the impact of the detailed report that is prepared and delivered to the clinician some weeks or months later is not made known to the pathologist. Pathologists occasionally publish their findings in a series of hospital autopsies, invariably showing that the clinical diagnoses and causes of death were incorrect in a significant proportion of cases. This diagnostic error rate may be relevant to the individual patient who may have been treated differently and with a different outcome if the correct diagnosis had been known in life. The correct diagnosis is also relevant for monitoring epidemiological trends of diseases. The cause of death may also be a crucially important end point in clinical trials of new therapies. The double-blind, randomised controlled clinical trial is regarded as the supreme tool of evidence-based medicine. Yet the information contained in the death certificate of a deceased trial participant may be wholly incorrect unless this was based upon autopsy data (Start et al., 1997).

The hospital autopsy continues to be of clinical importance, but mainly from the standpoint of clinical audit, which requires the analysis of large and unselected series of patients dying while under the care of a clinician. Yet autopsies have traditionally been centred on the circumstances of individual patients, and today's autopsy is very much a matter of happenchance, depending on the interest of the clinician and the willingness of the next of kin to grant permission. With the inevitable development of user-pays transactions in which the clinician chooses to pay for an autopsy from a fixed budget, one wonders if such a costly procedure will be rejected in favour of an alternative therapeutic option on behalf of a live patient. Clearly, if autopsy is perceived primarily as a means of achieving clinical audit, which is probably a correct view, then its practice is more a concern for hospital or health administrators than for individual clinicians with their inadequate budgets.

Clinical audit is of very great importance, yet it generally fails to ignite the interest of either clinicians or pathologists. Furthermore, audit is without value unless it is accompanied by appropriate modification and improvement in clinical practice. Without the strong support of the major stakeholders of the activity it is unlikely that hospital or health administrators will seek to invest the diminishing health budget in the development of a systematic and stand-ardised approach to hospital autopsy. Some institutions, however, have encouraged audit through the establishment of 'mortality meetings' in which all the hospital deaths in a preced-ing period are discussed openly. This exercise will obviously encourage autopsy practice as deaths can hardly be discussed adequately without a postmortem examination. Such meet-ings work well when the intention is to learn and modify behaviour as opposed to apportion blame or threaten legal action. Indeed a legalistic environment would lead to cover-ups, self-deception and a lowering of standards. Those institutions that support clinical audit of this kind will generally be the centres of medical excellence.

MODERN INDICATIONS FOR HOSPITAL AUTOPSY

It must be emphasised that apart from the issues of medicolegality, teaching and clinical audit, the autopsy remains a highly desirable if not mandatory activity (only forensic autop-sies are mandatory under law) within certain groups of subjects. These include patients suspected of dying of communicable diseases that are of major public concern, especially new and poorly understood diseases such as the human equivalent of bovine spongiform encephalopathy (mad cow disease), for which it is important to establish the true incidence, trends over time and lifestyle associations (epidemiology).

Another group of subjects that may lend itself to postmortem examination comprises those suffering from inherited disorders for which an accurate diagnosis will be of major concern to close relatives. Most of these diseases are rare and many are associated with prolonged suffering by both patient and family. In these situations the family and indeed the patient may be anxious that an autopsy be undertaken, not only because of the issue of possible inheritance but also as a contribution to medical knowledge for the benefit of others.

A third group are the patients for whom the cause of death is undeniably natural but only partly explicable. This is often true in the case of the elderly, but then the autopsy may only disclose a catalogue of minor problems with no clear-cut underlying cause. This type of autopsy assumes greater importance when death is judged to be premature as well as puz-zling, and the procedure clearly represents an attempt to uncover a significant but missed diagnosis.

The final group comprises patients who have received extensive medical or surgical treat-ment before death, but not sufficiently close to death to raise any medicolegal concerns. In requesting the autopsy, the clinician may wish to learn of the efficacy or unsuspected compli-cations of the treatment.

Individuals in each of the preceding categories may die in their own homes or in sites without autopsy facilities. The increasing trend towards dying in surroundings other than a major hospital poses logistic difficulties in all countries, since publicly funded systems to transport bodies to an appropriate site for an autopsy examination and budgets to cover the costs of the procedure itself do not exist. This is particularly frustrating for general practition-ers. Since a general practitioner may have had a longstanding professional relationship with a deceased patient, this concern may extend also to patients dying in hospital who do not have an autopsy.

The potential usefulness of a hospital autopsy will not be realised if the pathologist is not fully aware of the subject's clinical background, is inexperienced, or fails to slant the examination and final report towards the resolution of the underlying problems. Proper care in the achievement of an autopsy is dutiful and is the practical demonstration of respect for the deceased patient and the patient's family. Regrettably, adequate communication between pathologist and attending clinician is often lacking and the pathologist is often inexperienced. This lack of experience reflects the diminishing numbers of autopsies and the fact that they are frequently performed by trainees with little supervision. Examination boards worldwide insist that pathology trainees undertake a required number of autopsies. This is often achieved by the conduct of forensic autopsies which are more numerous than hospital autopsies, but pose different sets of problems.

FORENSIC AUTOPSIES

Forensic atuopsies are preformed when the cause of death is unknown or occurs under unnatural circumstances. The degree to which hospital and forensic autopsies differ is remarkable, but the distinction is not generally understood. Even the medical profession may be confused about the distinction. In many countries these different types of autopsy are regulated by different legislation, the UK, for example, has a 'Human Tissue Act' for hospital autopsy and a 'Coroner's Act' for forensic autopsy. The coroner (or equivalent) is legally but not necessarily medically trained and does not generally see, let alone examine, the body (the Medical Examiner system in America is different in this respect). The coroner has absolute authority to insist upon an autopsy and also to compel a medical practitioner (not necessarily a pathologist) to undertake the examination. Often the dissection will be performed by a pathologist with forensic training, but in rural areas the prosector may sometimes be a general practitioner. The stringency of this system was designed to ensure the protection of the interests of society under law. The individual instructed to perform the autopsy serves as a completely independent medical adviser to the coroner, explaining the mode of death in appropriate terms and being paid a fee for this service. When the death is natural, as it will be in a high proportion of cases, there is usually an obvious single explanation for what was a sudden and unexpected event. The procedure is therefore quick and straightforward. At the other extreme are the complex homicides requiring a detailed examination and sifting of forensic evidence that may take weeks to complete.

Because forensic autopsies are numerous and often involve healthy, young individuals dying under accidental circumstances, they provide opportunities for research, for the sampling of tissues for transplantation and surgical training. These practices are widespread but in most countries permitted only with the authorisation of the next of kin (which applies even when the deceased is registered as an organ donor).

DONATIONS

Some individuals decide to donate their bodies for medical research. Donation of bodies for the purpose of anatomical dissection by medical students is regulated by an 'Anatomy Act' or its equivalent (e.g. *Anatomy Act 1984* in the UK) and poses no administrative problems. Donation for medical research is more problematic unless it is linked to a specific ethically approved research program that includes facilities for the transport of bodies to a mortuary.

(Brain banks are also important for research into chronic neurological diseases such as Alzheimer's, Parkinson's and Huntington's diseases. Such donations also require the cooperation of the family.) When an individual forms the opinion that his or her disease is of unique importance, it is most unlikely that any donation can be made, except where a special system has been set up for the purpose.

Despite its long established position with western medical practice, autopsy examination is associated with difficulties of a religious, ethical, psychological, sociological, logistic, legal and economic nature. The benefits to humankind are multiple and very real, but are extremely difficult to evaluate and measure and the subject is one that most prefer not to discuss or contemplate. The development of national strategies to address the issues openly with a view to achieving consensus on lines of responsibility, standardisation of practice and funding mechanisms for hospital autopsies is probably a task that no government will choose to face in the foreseeable future. The practice will therefore stagger along as a relic of past tradition. But let it not be said that this complex sociological activity is driven by the morbid collective need of pathologists. If there were no requirement for, or benefit to be derived from postmortem examination the practice would cease immediately.

REFERENCES

Maulitz, R C. (1993) The pathological tradition. In *Companion Encyclopedia of the History of Medicine*, volume 1, edited by W.F. Bynum & R. Porter, pp. 169–191. London and New York: Routledge.

Start, R.D., Bury, J.P., Strachan, A.G. & Cross, S.S. (1997) Underwood JCE. Evaluating the reliability of causes of death in published clinical research. *Br Med J*, **314**, 271.

Further reading

Start, R.D. & Cotton, D.W.K. (1997) The current status of the autopsy. In *Progress in Pathology*, volume 3, edited by N. Kirkham & N.R. Lemoine, pp. 179–188. Edinburgh: Churchill Livingstone.

6

EDUCATIONAL ROLE OF PATHOLOGY

Altogether they teach in academies far too many things, and far too much that is useless. Then the individual professors extend their departments too much — far beyond the wants of their hearers. In former days lectures were read in chemistry and botany as belonging to medicine, and the physician could manage them. Now, both these have become so extensive that each of them requires a life; yet acquaintance with both is expected from the physician. Nothing can come of this; one thing must be neglected or forgotten for the sake of the other

Johann von Goethe in *Conversations with Eckermann* (1823–1832)

The more you know, the less you understand

Tao Te Ching

How much pathology does one need to know?

PATHOLOGY FOR PROFESSIONS

Generally speaking, anatomical pathologists (regardless of whether they are employed by universities, hospital authorities or private companies, or are self-employed) represent a subspecialty group within the medical profession. The term profession implies an organisation which offers a service that is founded on a body of knowledge, skills, attitudes and ethical codes that has developed over many years, indeed centuries. Another feature of a profession is that it is self-regulating. Part of this self-regulation includes the imparting of knowledge, skills and attitudes to future members of the profession, to trainee specialists within the profession and, within the framework of continuing medical education, to all those in active practice. The Hippocratic oath makes teaching an obligation. Since pathology is the study of disease, it is evident that pathologists must play a large role in medical education.

Educational commitments do not end with the medical profession. The cause and nature of disease is relevant to the practice of nursing, dentistry, physiotherapy, occupational therapy, veterinary science and forensic science. With the jostling and manoeuvring within the tertiary education sector for the purposes of attracting students in larger and larger numbers, courses providing instruction in pathology are now being offered in university science faculties across the globe. This policy has been driven more by economic expedience than by educational need. The mismatch between the number of medically trained academic pathologists and the number of students learning about pathology is already evident and will increase.

Human pathology is relatively meaningless as an isolated discipline. Histology, gross anatomy, genetics, embryology, molecular biology, microbiology, physiology and biochemistry are prerequisites for an understanding of disordered structure and function. Pathology must also be correlated with the clinical disciplines to imbue it with practical meaning. Without these prerequisites standards of learning are undermined and without the clinical correlation the relevance of the discipline diminishes. Pathology taught out of context descends to mere rote learning. During his conversations with Eckermann, Johann von Goethe remarked: 'We retain from our studies only that which we practically apply'.

TEACHING METHODS FOR MEDICAL STUDENTS AND STUDENTS OF THE ALLIED HEALTH PROFESSIONS

Anatomical pathology is an intensely visual discipline and as such its teaching is visually based. In a lecture, the lecturer is often eclipsed by the projected images of diseased tissues and is more a demonstrator aiming to develop the observational skills of the audience and explain how disordered structure correlates with symptoms and signs of disease. This, however, is no longer the dominant format for teaching pathology to students.

The subject matter of pathology education in medical schools can be divided into general pathology and systemic pathology. General pathology deals with the various categories of disease, explaining the causes and mechanisms that underlie disease processes such as microbial infection, arterial occlusion, or cancer. Systemic pathology describes the disease entities that may be found in each system of the body: respiratory, cardiovascular, nervous system and so on. Whilst an understanding of the major categories of diseases and their underlying mechanisms is essential if the practice of medicine is to be scientifically based, a system-by-system approach to the teaching of anatomical pathology that is not integrated with other disciplines is outmoded.

It is extraordinary how old habits die hard, especially within a profession that is prone towards conservatism. The move away from system-based teaching of pathology (conducted in isolation) is rather like the ending of a ritual that has been performed in one's family for centuries. No longer are pathologists permitted to describe weird and fascinating diseases to excite feelings of prurience in their audience. However, the demise of the black humour factor is not the manifestation of mere political correctness. Rather it is the realisation that disease and death are inherently fascinating subjects (as indicated by the content of television programs), but that one's business should be rightfully driven by educational need rather than the desire to encourage morbid curiosity in oneself or others.

THE NEEDS OF THE MEDICAL STUDENT

The needs of the medical student have rarely been defined, and most medical students report that their medical education did not prepare them for life on the wards. And despite the traditional abundance of pathology teaching, the emergent doctor has always had a limited awareness of the role of laboratory medicine in the management of disease. Indeed, much of the content of the first part this book will be unfamiliar to the medical profession. What are the needs of the junior doctor in relation to the discipline of pathology? They are to:

1. understand and explain the basic mechanisms underlying the major disease processes,
2. use knowledge of pathological principles in order to formulate possible diagnoses on the basis of a patient's history and findings on clinical examination,
3. know when and how to request a laboratory investigation including an autopsy examination,
4. understand the significance of a result or report that comes back from the laboratory,
5. explain the result or report to a patient when so authorised.

It is fair to state that the traditional teaching of pathology has not been slanted towards the achievement of these five learning objectives. The main problem has been the attempt to teach pathology out of clinical context. Medical schools have solved the dilemma by the introduction of either integrated teaching or problem-based learning. Both teaching methods are heavily resource dependent and require major adjustments in teaching styles.

Integrated teaching necessitates coordinated input by two or (generally) more disciplines. For example, a lesson on breast cancer may involve a panel that includes a pathologist, a radiologist, an epidemiologist, a surgeon and an advocate for women's health. A successful and balanced presentation will occur only through the dedication of a panel leader combined with the good will and expertise of the group. However, trying to organise clinicians or academics into providing a coordinated and balanced program has been likened to an attempt at herding cats, and clinicians will sometimes state that they can teach everything that needs to be known about a particular subject by themselves. Integrated teaching may also suffer from being excessively didactic. Problem-based learning, on the other hand, implies a self-directed approach to the acquisition of knowledge (Schmidt, 1993). Problems are generally built on clinical scenarios that are relevant to the practice of medicine. Students are given limited amounts of information such as they would gain from interviewing and observing a patient. Working as a group, they categorise the information and develop hypotheses that would explain what they have heard and seen. If the problem has been constructed well, the students will formulate their own learning objectives relevant to the problem. Considerable care must be given to the development of problems that will yield learning objectives that are achievable given prior levels of knowledge. In the beginning of a medical course, the problems will need to trigger learning objectives that relate to normal structure, function and behaviour, with disease mechanisms entering in measured steps. Students need to be given generic learning objectives, such as the five listed above, to ensure that their specific learning objectives are congruent with the long-term goals of the course. With problem-based learning, students are exposed to relatively little didactic teaching, but the facilitators of problem-based tutorials require special skills for working with groups as well as having an all-round medical knowledge to ensure that the students remain focused. Students learning in this way build up a knowledge base slowly, but retain information when it is linked to a practical problem (Bosman, 1996; Benbow et al., 1996).

Some of the traditional teaching methods adopted by anatomical pathologists are beginning to recede into the mists of yesteryear. The demise of the hospital autopsy is discussed in Chapter 5. A medical student can obtain little benefit from attending an autopsy unless the demonstration of diseased organs is carefully correlated with clinical history. Unfortunately, the procedure is rarely associated with comprehensive clinical input and the most the student can expect to gain from the experience is an appreciation of the appearance of diseased tissue, as well as normal anatomical relationships. This may be achieved more conveniently by a visit to a pathology museum. Museums are also in a state of decline because of the expense of maintaining potted specimens and the increasing demands on medical school space through the growth of other disciplines. It is nevertheless important that medical students understand why autopsies are performed (see Chapter 5) and know how the structure of an organ or tissue becomes altered through a disease process, as well as the underlying mechanisms involved.

LIMITATIONS OF DISEASE-BASED TEACHING

Most of the diseases mentioned in this text are serious and life-threatening. The disease-based or pathological approach to medical education encourages the doctor to interpret a patient's symptoms in the light of prior knowledge regarding the natural history of disease. If the symptoms cannot be related to a specific disease entity, it is not uncommon for doctors to disbelieve, dismiss or contradict the patient's view. If, on the other hand, a major underlying disease is suspected, the practitioner is likely to transmit uncertainty or ambiguity to the patient until the final or working diagnosis is achieved. The underlying mechanisms may be forgotten or deemed too complicated to explain to the patient in the limited time available (despite the traditional role of the healer as an interpreter of symptoms), and the prognosis may be given in accurate statistical terms that are incomprehensible to the patient.

The vast majority of symptoms that occur in an individual's lifetime relate to factors other than major or life-threatening diseases. Most consultations in the general or family practitioner setting centre on such minor or self-limiting complaints and the same minor problems will surface in the hospital setting. The manner in which such symptoms are handled is in part the result of disease-based teaching and explains why both patients and an increasing proportion of family practitioners have adopted complementary or alternative approaches to health care. Not only does the alternative practitioner accept the patient's symptoms at face value, but he/she also operates in an unrushed and non-depersonalised environment that provides continuity of care and time to empathise with the patient's predicament. Furthermore, the alternative practitioner will generally explain the symptoms on the basis of a very simple and therefore intelligible mechanism (e.g. Candida infection, minor vertebral misalignment, etc.), and offer hope in the form of a reliable, non-toxic remedy involving the full participation of the patient (Buckman & Sabbagh, 1993).

The disease-based approach to medical education is just one of the factors that has made the patient feel like a product on the shelf of a supermarket–labelled, packaged and handled impersonally. By contrast, complementary or alternative medicine offers the patient the choices available to the consumers in the supermarket (Buckman & Sabbagh, 1993). The question is whether the consumer has enough knowledge and experience to make an informed choice. Fortunately, most symptoms are not harbingers of a dangerous underlying disease and the alternative practitioner will at worst do no harm, but very likely alleviate suffering by a combination of psychological and placebo effects. The danger arises when either an alternative or a conventional practitioner fails to act on a symptom or sign that calls for urgent investigation and treatment or offers hope (a two-edged sword) inappropriately.

THE STUDENT–TEACHER RELATIONSHIP

The student–teacher relationship is a topic that has been neglected, particularly with respect to the teaching of pathology. The student–teacher relationship should presage a good patient–doctor relationship. These relationships may overlap when teaching is performed at the bedside. Whilst the pathologist may not teach in the presence of a living patient, teaching should nevertheless exemplify good interpersonal skills. These include not only the effective communication of relevant clinical knowledge, but the willingness to listen to, understand and address student concerns. Students are not merely empty vessels that require filling, but are responsive and responsible individuals with different needs, interests and social backgrounds.

Naturally the continuous, one-to-one doctor–patient relationship cannot be recapitulated at the student–teacher level. Indeed, in a modern integrated medical course, a pathologist may deliver a smattering of lectures throughout the entire course, rather than a complete series within a stand-alone academic subject. In a problem-based (essentially patient-based) course, the pathologist has the opportunity to serve as a role model in a problem-based tutorial setting, even if such tutoring involves knowledge, skills and attitudes beyond the traditional confines of pathology. Like the patient, the student enrolled in a problem-based course has a 'problem'. The resources offered by a pathology department must be slanted towards the resolution of this specific problem and not other unrelated or vaguely related problems. Forcing irrelevant teaching upon students will be as counterproductive as giving patients the wrong treatment.

The preceding comments might appear to diminish the once central role of the pathologist in medical education. Yet it must be emphasised that pathology underpins the acquisition of interpersonal skills (as well as knowledge), including the same desirable skills that alternative practitioners have retained and conventional practitioners have discarded. Adherents of conventional medical practice need not be reticent about the vast body of knowledge on disease mechanisms or the complex processes that must be followed to reach a correct diagnosis. The challenge is to render the concealed areas of medical practice transparent, simple and accessible to the patient. This should not be done merely through the media, but in the direct experiential context of the doctor–patient relationship. The credibility of conventional medicine relies heavily on the hidden work of the pathologist, and the responsibility of imparting this realisation to medical students and ultimately to patients will fall increasingly on the broader community of medical educationalists.

TEACHING PATHOLOGY AT POSTGRADUATE LEVEL

Selected aspects of teaching that were once part of the congested medical school curriculum are now taught more appropriately at a later stage of clinical training. Radiologists, for example, need a very practical understanding of both normal and diseased structure if they are to interpret images correctly. Oncologists must be thoroughly versed in the pathology of cancer. Surgeons have to recognise disease that they encounter during operations. Gastroenterologists need to recognise and understand the natural history of disease that they discover during the endoscopic examination of a colon or stomach. All clinicians need to make effective use of laboratory medicine. Apart from any formal teaching of these groups, teaching occurs in a less formal setting during regular clinicopathological meetings (see Chapter 4).

Teaching and training must also occur within the discipline of anatomical pathology, both for trainees (see Chapter 2) and in the form of continuing medical education for those in practice. Continuing education is coordinated through both national and international organisations that promote meetings lasting from one day to a week. These organisations may also sponsor journals that publish articles of an educational nature. There are at least one dozen refereed journals that are directly relevant to the practice of anatomical pathology. They are published monthly or quarterly and each issue contains about ten articles. Anatomical pathologists participate in continuing education not merely by attending meetings and reading journals but in a more dynamic sense by contributing to both.

The anatomical pathologist has a central role in medical education, supporting learning at many levels and on behalf of multiple disciplines with particular specialised needs. Perhaps the most important vehicle for ensuring uniformly high standards of education and practice across the globe is the textbook supported by specialist journals.

REFERENCES

Benbow, E.W., Rutinhauser, S., Stoddart, R.W., Andrew, S.M. & Freemont, A.J. (1996) Pathologists and problem-based learning. *J Pathol*, **180**, 340–342.

Bosman, F.T. (1996) New curricula. *J Pathol*, **180**, 346–348.

Buckman, R. & Sabbagh, K. (1993) *Magic or Medicine? An Investigation into Healing.* London: Macmillan.

Schmidt, H.G. (1993) Foundations of problem-based learning: some explanatory notes. *Med Educ,* **27**, 422-432.

von Goethe, J. W. (1984) *Conversations with Eckermann (1823–1832).* San Francisco: North Point Press.

7

PATHOLOGY AND RESEARCH

*It is only our individual weakness which makes us satisfied
with what has been discovered by others*

Michel de Montaigne

How does the pathologist advance medical research?

CLINICAL RESEARCH

How do the specific attributes of the discipline of anatomical pathology lend themselves to
the advance of medical research? The most general contribution has been to the systematic
classification of disease known as nosology. This process begins with the arrangement of
the many thousands of known diseases into logical groupings, rather like the phylogenetic
classification of species of animals and plants. Diseases may be grouped according to the
usual age, sex or race of affected subjects, by the part of the body that is most severely
affected, or by the type of treatment that would be employed. Although such classifications
might have some use, they all fail to place diseases within distinct, non-overlapping boundaries. To achieve a more meaningful approach to nosology, it is necessary to look at the
fundamental nature of a disease, specifically the mechanisms underlying its causation (aetiology) and evolution (pathogenesis).

Through the pioneering work of Rudolf Virchow (see Chapter 1) diseases that may be
grouped generically as disorders of growth (of which cancer would be the most lethal example) came to be linked through a mechanism involving dysfunction of growth control at the
level of the cell. However, Virchow's inductive thinking (his attempt to derive an underlying
rule from multiple observations) turned out to be too all-embracing. The principle of cellular
disturbance as the basis of all disease collapsed with the recognition that a large group of
diseases was caused by the invasion of the body by micro-organisms. Further inductive
reasoning led to the grouping of disorders of growth into a subcategory called neoplasms:
masses characterised by progressive and autonomous increase in size. Those neoplasms
that remained localised were called benign and those with the potential for distant spread
were called malignant (Willis, 1952). Further classification of neoplasms was then based upon
the underlying type of tissue (see Chapter 22). For example benign neoplasms composed of
glandular (secretory) tissue were termed adenomas. Dukes (1930) described all the small

mushroom-like growths (often called polyps) that might occur in the colon as adenomas. Morson (1962) observed the various types of colonic polyp carefully and applied the principles governing the properties of a neoplasm to the various subtypes. By this process of deductive reasoning, Morson split the 'adenomas' into three groups: genuine adenomas, hyperplastic polyps (simple overgrowths) and malformations. He also emphasised that as neoplasms, adenomas would not only increase in size progressively, but had the potential to develop into cancer. It is now accepted that most cancers of the colon arise from preexisting adenomas and that the two lesions represent a neoplastic continuum from benign to malignant.

The contribution of anatomical pathology to the recognition and classification of disease has come about through the processes of inductive and deductive reasoning applied to naked-eye and microscopic observations of diseased organs and tissues. Anatomical pathologists are responsible for the initial detailed description and classification of virtually every structural abnormality that may occur in the human body. These morphological descriptions are of limited value unless they are linked in a comprehensive manner to clinical observations. The latter include the age, gender and race of the patient, social and occupational history as well as the signs, symptoms, complications and outcome of the particular disorder producing the morphological change.

Given the large number of disease characteristics, it is necessary to identify cardinal diagnostic criteria. The most fundamental of all will be the cause or aetiology of the disease. This is straightforward for some categories of disease for which there is a single, well-defined cause. The best example of this type of category would be those infectious diseases in which a specific micro-organism produces a highly characteristic disease course, as occurs in mumps, measles or chicken pox. In the case of the benign and malignant neoplasms, classification is based partly on the clinical behaviour of a growth and partly on its morphological characteristics. Neoplasms present a vast range of appearances and the initial approach to nomenclature has generally been one of splitting into finer and finer variants. Useful meaning comes from this approach when it is shown that two similar but nevertheless distinguishable variants differ in their clinical behaviour or response to treatment. By splitting variants in this way, one is in effect defining a new type of disease. Pathological literature includes innumerable types of neoplasms that were split from a former category by the process of careful observation, clinical correlation and deductive reasoning.

Eventually, however, the deductive application of simple sets of rules must give way to the higher cognitive function represented by inductive reasoning. Based upon a particular underlying principle, it might be hypothesised that several types of neoplasm in fact belong to a 'family'. This general principle will usually relate to an area of basic biomedical knowledge. For example, a group of neoplasms arising in all manner of sites appeared to be characterised by hormonal function, similar microscopic features, particular biochemical pathways and a common embryological origin. The group was bracketed together as APUDoma (Amine Precursor Uptake and Decarboxylation) (Pearse 1969). Although these tumours are still conceived as a 'family', the underlying premises for their categorisation turned out to be only partially correct. Different diseases may also be grouped when they are observed to occur together more frequently than one might expect on the basis of their occurrence in the general population. The coincidence of two or more diseases in one individual and/or in a single family constitutes a syndrome. When a family is involved, the syndrome is likely to be inherited. Anatomical pathologists have recognised new syndromes with the aid of the powerful dimension of microscopic analysis. This has been achieved through the study of both surgical specimens (Williams, 1965) and autopsy examination (Beckwith, 1969).

The recognition of both diseases and syndromes requires not only careful clinicopathological correlation but also the demonstration of a similar pattern of pathology and clinical behaviour in a large series of patients. Confidence in the existence of a new disease or syndrome will increase when similar findings are reported by others. When the findings have been replicated a sufficient number of times, a disease or syndrome assumes a mantle of respectability, even though the underlying cause may be unknown. Diseases that are diagnosed by the presence of structural change have been documented in meticulous detail in medical literature. The contribution of anatomical pathologists to the recognition and classification of new diseases and the establishment of diagnostic criteria encapsulates the unique and fundamental contribution of the discipline to clinical research. Furthermore, this approach establishes pathological diagnosis as an exercise that is evidence based. This contrasts with the therapeutic arm of medical practice that is based primarily upon the results of observation alone (empiricism).

The type of research described above is different from most people's concept of biomedical research. It occurs in hospitals or university departments of pathology linked to hospitals and springs directly from the routine practice of diagnostic anatomical pathology. The costs are low compared to those of biomedical research because one is not undertaking multiple experiments requiring expensive reagents and laboratory equipment. The prerequisites are good laboratory systems (see Chapter 3), ready access to medical literature, the support of clinical colleagues and a flair for clinical research. Naturally one is not going to discover the cure for cancer, but treatment of cancer is only one side of the coin. Diagnosis is the basis on which treatment is founded, yet correct diagnosis of disease is generally, and at times mistakenly, taken for granted.

BIOMEDICAL RESEARCH

Despite the importance of the contribution to research made by anatomical pathology, is there an argument for placing the period of active research in the past and suggesting that the discipline has matured and lost its former academic relevance, now serving merely as a diagnostic service? Clearly the focus of biomedical research has moved towards the reductionism of molecular biology. The drive to discover a new disease has been replaced by the exhilaration of being the first to clone and characterise a new gene. Unravelling the genome and constructing step by step the complex cascades of signalling pathways that orchestrate normal cellular function is an essential prerequisite for a full understanding of diseases that are cellular in origin (such as cancer). Nevertheless, the time has come when molecular mechanisms at the cellular level must be correlated with pathological changes at the level of tissues. In other words, while the traditional task of correlating clinical and pathological observations may have come close to completion, the next major challenge is molecular–pathological–clinical correlation.

Some of the ways in which anatomical pathology will assist in the translation of advances at the molecular level are already apparent. Anatomical pathologists have been using monoclonal antibodies to study molecular signatures for 15 years (see Chapters 3 and 22). Once new genes are cloned and sequenced, the protein products of those genes can be synthesised artificially and used to generate 'second generation' monoclonal antibodies (Xing et al., 1992). These can be used to localise the protein products and determine whether they are expressed in the nucleus, cytoplasm or cell membrane of normal and diseased cells. This assists in uncovering the function of a gene and demonstrating its involvement in disease processes. Using microdissection techniques assisted by lasers it is possible to excise small groups of cells or even single cells from a tissue section, extract the DNA and screen it for genetic mutations (Emmert-Buck et al., 1996). This provides a direct link between the structural basis of cancer evolution and the underlying genetic alterations. From a specimen of cancer it is possible to sample cells representing the various steps in the evolutionary progression of the malignancy (see Chapter 24) and build up a corresponding sequence of genetic changes. Such knowledge will assist in developing an understanding of cancer causation and in formulating novel treatment strategies. In research of this kind, the trained eye and clinical knowledge of the anatomical pathologist provides a conduit between the world of molecules and the level of the whole patient.

Interestingly, new molecular findings are beginning to challenge many traditional views on disease classification. Morson's separation of colonic 'adenomas' into bona fide benign neoplasms versus simple overgrowths (hyperplastic polyps) (see above) is now negated by the demonstration that hyperplastic polyps, like neoplasms, appear to originate from a single cell driven by a genetic mutation (Williams, 1997). The genetic change in fact leads to the conversion of a proto-oncogene into an oncogene (called K-*ras*), one of the genes implicated in the evolution of colon cancer (see Chapter 23). This is just one example of new insights that will revolutionise our thinking on the nature of disease.

Clinical research flows naturally from the work of the anatomical pathologist in which tissue specimens are studied with well-tried techniques and stored in files for future analysis (see Chapter 3). Biomedical research has now developed a large and independent momentum and uses methodologies that are powerful but have little relevance to the routine work of the hospital anatomical pathologist. It is clear that collaboration of anatomical pathology and basic biomedical science is required if the next step in the evolution of anatomical pathology is to be fully realised. The sophisticated tools of the molecular biologist need to be aligned with the eye of the anatomical pathologist in order to facilitate the translation of basic insight obtained by studying the machinery of the cell into advances in the clinical management of disease.

REFERENCES

Beckwith, J.B. (1969) Macroglossia, omphalocele, adrenal cytomegaly, gigantism and hyperplastic visceromegaly. *Birth Defects*, **5**, 188–196.

Dukes, C.E. (1930) The hereditary factor in polyposis intestini, or multiple adenomata. *The Cancer Rev*, **5**, 241–251.

Emmert-Buck, M.R., Bonner, R.F., Smith, P.D., Chuaqui, R.F., Zhuang, Z., Goldstein, S.R., Weiss, R.A. & Liotta, L.A. (1996) Laser capture microdissection. *Science* 1996, **274**, 998–1001.

Morson, B.C. (1962) Some peculiarities in the histology of intestinal polyps. *Dis Colon Rectum*, **5**, 337–344.

Pearse, A.G.E. (1969) The cytochemistry and ulstrastructure of polypeptide hormone-producing cells of the APUD series, and the embryologic, physiologic and pathologic implications of the concept. *J Histochem Cytochem*, **17**, 303–313.

Williams, E.D. (1965) A review of 17 cases of carcinoma of the thyroid and phaeochromocytomas. *J Clin Pathol*, **18**, 288–292.

Williams, G.T. (1997) Metaplastic (hyperplastic) polyps of the large bowel: benign neoplasms after all? *Gut,* **40**, 691–692.

Willis, R.A. (1952) *The Spread of Tumours in the Human Body.* London: Butterworth and Co.

Xing, P.X., Prenzoska, J., Layton, G.T., Devine, P.L. & McKenzie, I.F.C. (1992) Second generation monoclonal antibodies to intestinal MUC2 peptide reactive with colon cancer. *J Natl Cancer Inst*, **84**, 699–703.

— 8 —

THE AGE OF ECONOMIC REALISM

*O miserable race of man! Of how many objects you make
yourself the slave for the sake of monetary gain*

Leonardo da Vinci

Should pathology survive as an academic discipline?

MODERN PATHOLOGY

Attitudes towards disease and its management have been moulded by various systems of thought operating through the ages. The present age is characterised by: (1) a preoccupation with information and its rapid and wide dissemination by electronic media, (2) genetic research, with its ramifying social and ethical implications, and (3) the relentless march of economic rationalisation. Pathology, once a hidden and protected kernel within the world of medicine, is now fully exposed to the forces of change.

The exponents of modern business practices place great value on mission statements, long term goals, specific objectives and strategic plans. These serve as shocks to accelerate adaptation and indeed permit survival in a rapidly changing world. Where does medicine and pathology in particular fit into all this? Pathology has certainly matured, but during a time-frame that can be measured in centuries if not millennia. The old has been rejected only after exhaustive testing of the new.

As discussed in Chapters 1 and 5, anatomical pathology was founded upon human dissection. Over the last few decades the autopsy has receded and histopathology (or surgical pathology) has become the dominant activity. Histopathology has continued to develop through the addition of technical refinements including histochemistry, electron microscopy, cytopathology, immunohistochemistry, static and flow cytometry and molecular technology. Parallel medical progress in the fields of endoscopy, flexible fibre-optic endoscopy, video-endoscopy and radiological imaging now allow diagnostic tissue samples to be collected with relative ease from any region of the body, obviating the requirement for invasive surgery.

The Harvard pathologist William Councilman (1854–1933) noted the central role of pathology laboratories within hospitals, by which means 'the study of tissues or fluids from individual cases' could be carried out, as well as 'the study of questions concerning disease'

(Maulitz, 1993). The latter comment relates to research. Although the term pathology can be equated with the entire range of laboratory medicine, including its diagnostic and research arms, some would regard such a viewpoint as unacceptable and historically inexact. Pathological chemistry, microbiology and experimental pathology (essentially the study of disease with the aid of animals) developed as quite independent disciplines that have at times converged with or become bracketed with anatomical pathology. For example, the separate laboratory diagnostic disciplines of anatomical pathology, microbiology, chemical pathology and haematology have often been closely linked in terms of geographical location, systems of administration and training and accreditation through professional organisations such as the Royal Colleges or American Boards. Experimental pathology and anatomical pathology have traditionally been close allies within university departments or institutes of pathology. However, the passage of time has always been accompanied by specialisation and the splintering of larger groupings into smaller units with common interests.

STRUCTURE OF ACADEMIC PATHOLOGY

In the past, the coupling of anatomical and experimental pathology generated large departmental empires within university-based medical schools that served as central powerhouses for both teaching and medical research. Experimental pathology encompassed not only animal-based research but also came to utilise techniques for the study of preparations of living cells of both human and animal origin as well as exploiting advances in biochemistry, immunology and molecular biology that could be applied to the study of human disease. Gradually, however, other more clinical disciplines such as medicine and surgery began to foster research of a similar kind, which would today be called biomedical research rather than experimental pathology. Since research funds are always scarce and a large proportion is earmarked for research into human disease, non-clinical university departments (primarily established for the study of normal structure and function and research into molecular and cellular biology), have also moved into the field of biomedical research. This broadening of the research base has resulted in a similar broadening of the teaching base.

Departments of pathology not only lost their monopoly to clinical and preclinical university departments, but also found themselves in competition with independent biomedical research institutes, in which scientists may focus their attention exclusively on research without distractions in the form of undergraduate teaching or clinical responsibility. In this way, the small beginnings of experimental pathology have expanded into a colossal industry. However, through this process of generalising human disease-based research, much of the early source of strength underlying the discipline of pathology has been sapped. Nevertheless, university or hospital-based pathology departments remain as the traditional bases for receiving human tissues and diagnosing disease by the examination of such specimens. The blend of clinical, anatomical and technical skills that is contained within the discipline means that it is still able to make further important and unique contributions to medical research.

COMMERCIAL PATHOLOGY

We should not take the totally negative view of commercialisation as merely an attitude that seeks to generate maximum profit from a transaction. Rather we should look at the issue of accountability with respect to the provision of a service. The economic rationalists have deemed that western medicine is not merely expensive but wastefully so. This has been shown by evidence based on health outcomes research (Gray, 1997). The inevitable financial restructuring is already impacting upon pathology as well as other branches of medicine. Pathology is particularly vulnerable to the forces of economic rationalisation, but also has a number of innate strengths.

One feature of pathology is a relative ignorance of its role (on the part of both health professionals and the public) as compared with those of the more therapeutic activities of the clinical disciplines. At the same time, laboratories have well-developed information systems allowing tests to be costed out accurately. It is therefore not surprising that many diagnostic laboratories have been converted into business units. This has in turn necessitated the separation of the traditional arms of research, teaching and practice in order to cost out the various activities individually. This is fine so long as separation is followed by reintegration. Unfortunately, the reintegration is currently lagging behind.

WHO IS THE CUSTOMER?

If pathology is a business with the pathologist as the provider, then who is the customer? Although the principle of payment by an informed user might appear to be consistent with current economic thought, the process of health rationalisation has deemed that pathology should become a clinical support service, with the client or customer focus shifting from the patient to the doctor treating the patient. This means that the final decision about how a specimen is examined or even if is examined at all is made by neither the pathologist nor by the subject from whom the sample was taken, but by the doctor treating the patient. Since doctors increasingly have to work within fixed budgets, they will naturally be tempted to prioritise purchases and opt for the most cost-effective buy. So even those pathologists who are the most critical in their practice, the most meticulous in following internationally agreed standardised protocols, who are continually applying new and clinically beneficial scientific knowledge to their work, who are actively engaged in teaching and research and who have taken the trouble to develop special diagnostic skills, are now also required to demonstrate that their work practices are cost effective.

The commercialisation of pathology is not merely a future challenge but is happening now. The commercial attitude risks the exchange of professional and scientific integrity for monetary gain, and no sector, public or private, is immune from this attitude. The problems posed by converting pathology tests into commodities that can be purchased relate to the costing of the test and the awareness of the purchaser of the need for the test and its interpretation. Let us consider these two issues.

Costing of tests

The costing of tests that are performed through mass automation is simple. Laboratories use the same or similar reagents, automatic analysers and employ staff on scales that will be common to a particular nation. Rent and services can be factored in to give an exact cost per specimen. If the automatic analysers are used day and night to their full capacity, a situation of maximum efficiency will be achieved relative to any rival laboratory. The tests conducted by an anatomical pathologist are different since each specimen needs to be individually described, dissected, processed, sectioned, stained and examined microscopically. Corners can be cut at each one of these steps to save money. Those organisations that aim for the highest standards of health care will be the least likely to cut corners, but they must now furnish evidence that their activities are effective insofar as they translate into meaningful clinical outcomes.

The current professional structuring of pathology services often results in low-volume, high-intensity, low-profit anatomical pathology being bracketed with high-volume, low-intensity, high-profit fully automated laboratory testing (particularly chemical pathology and haematology). The more commercially driven organisations may wish to accept anatomical pathology specimens in order to enhance the goodwill factor that exists between customer (clinician) and provider (pathologist), as this may encourage the submission of more profitable types of test sample. The loss engendered by anatomical pathology can be reduced by cutting corners or cross-subsidisation, but will in any event be more than offset by the more profitable forms of testing. One method of cost cutting is to limit the provision of special investigations such as electron microscopy, immunohistochemistry and autopsy, thereby making competitors who offer a comprehensive service appear relatively expensive. When the full costing of anatomical pathology testing as performed in centres of excellence is compared with commercial costing, the difference may be considerable. The marketplace philosophy was created to deal with unproductive businesses that would collapse when placed in competition with more efficient organisations. However, effectiveness relates to both cost and quality. In other words, good management and professional integrity are independent characteristics, but must work together harmoniously in order to generate true cost-effectiveness.

Consumer awareness

The marketplace philosophy assumes that the purchaser knows exactly what he or she wants and will simply shop around until a vendor is found offering the cheapest buy and fastest delivery service. These are the only issues: knowing what is wanted, cost and speed. However, a good pathology report costs more and takes longer than a bad report. This would not matter if surgeons, for example, could always tell a good product from a bad one. Good pathology attempts to align the best of modern scientific and medical knowledge to the needs of the patient, and such knowledge may be highly relevant to a third party such as an oncologist who may be required to treat the patient with chemotherapy or radiotherapy following surgery. The surgeon may be perfectly happy with a pathological report, yet the same report may be unhelpful to the oncologist. Unfortunately, there is usually no going back, and the patient may be offered treatment (or not) on the basis of inadequate information. When there is the possibility of revisiting a specimen that has been inadequately reported, the time required for this task is often greater than that required to do the job properly in the first place.

The preceding scenario is not unusual and illustrates the fallacy of the marketplace philosophy taken to its extreme. The good pathologist views neither the surgeon nor the oncologist as the customer, but seeks to do his or her best on behalf of the patient. This is the crucial issue. The energies of the pathologist are required both at diagnosis and at the point of translating a diagnosis into optimal patient management. The way forward is an old idea—pathologists need to focus on professional standards and patient outcomes.

TEACHING ANATOMICAL PATHOLOGY

Anatomical pathology comprises research, teaching and diagnostic service, each supporting and strengthening the others. We have considered two major challenges to the discipline: the commercialisation of service, and the wide generalisation of research into the mechanisms of disease which was once the relatively exclusive province of pathologists. The challenge to its traditional role in teaching is equally if not even more serious than the other two. Excellence in teaching has long-term benefits in the fields of both research and practice, and an understanding of disease is obviously essential for safety and competency in the practice of medicine. Medical school curricula are often driven by university politics and agendas that may be far removed from practical educational needs. In the Darwinian struggle for curricular survival, the once central position occupied by pathology in the medical school has been progressively eroded and replaced by newer basic science disciplines such as molecular biology, and the burgeoning social and behavioural sciences incorporating medical ethics and communication skills. An integrated approach to teaching may at one level appear to undermine the integrity of traditional disciplines (or departments), but on the other hand, a teacher in an integrated problem-based course must, by necessity, venture from the narrow confines of his or her own discipline. The growth of mutual understanding and respect that should flow from this process may in fact strengthen rather than weaken individual disciplines.

The approach adopted in this text has been to base the teaching of anatomical pathology on practice in a clinical context. An integrated approach has been encouraged by focusing on the interface between pathology with science, medicine and the humanities. In order to survive, a discipline must not only be of practical relevance in a rapidly changing world, but understood to be so. This is the central learning objective.

REFERENCES

Gray, M. (1997) *Evidence Based Health Policy*. Edinburgh: Churchill Livingstone.
Maulitz, R.C. (1993) The pathological tradition. In *Companion Encyclopedia of the History of Medicine,* volume 1, edited by W.F. Bynum & R. Porter., pp. 169–191. London and New York: Routledge,

Further reading

Mapstone, N. & Quirke, P. (1997) The pathologist in the 21st century: man or machine? In *Progress in Pathology*, volume 3, edited by N. Kirkham & N.R. Lemoine, N.R., pp. 139–151. Edinburgh: Churchill Livingstone.

9

OBSERVING AND DESCRIBING DISEASE

Strive when you go about to observe

Leonardo da Vinci

What is the educational benefit of studying diseased tissue?

SPECIMENS THAT MAY BE OBSERVED

This chapter introduces pathological terms that will be discussed in more detail in Parts II to V. The glossary will be of assistance, but the reader is advised to revisit this chapter after studying the remainder of the book.

Disease may be observed at the macroscopic level in the living patient, for example during clinical examination, surgery, endoscopy or through imaging modalities. More detailed inspection is possible in the case of dead tissue, whether this be at autopsy, in surgical cut-ups in the laboratory, museum specimens or static images. A complete and integrated perspective on the gross appearance of disease will be achieved in a sequence such as:

magnetic resonance imaging → surgery → dissection of surgical specimen
→ correlation with imaging and histology.

Another sequence might be:

echocardiogram → autopsy examination
→ correlation with histology and echocardiogram.

It is difficult to achieve such integration across multiple specialties and the issue is raised in order to contrast the richest possible learning experience with the valuable but much diminished opportunities for learning afforded by museum specimens or two-dimensional images in books or on computer screens. The following discussion centres upon the museum specimen or 'pot'.

The museum specimen has long been used to test the student or postgraduate trainee in specialties such as surgery, radiology, oncology and radiotherapy, as well as pathology. Such a specimen has three great advantages over the two-dimensional image: (1) it can be viewed from all sides; (2) size can be gauged without difficulty; (3) the specimen is real and can be correlated with the clinical history of the patient. It should also be stated, however, that the final appearance of the sliced, trimmed or dissected organ always represents a distortion of the 'truth'. Apart from the fact that the specimen is generally anaemic and cannot be palpated or dissected by the observer, it represents a 'classic' or 'textbook' appearance, which is not necessarily the presentation encountered in routine clinical practice. The classic appearances of disease processes can be learned in the same way that we learn to recognise the various makes of car, species of bird or paintings by the great masters. Such a skill will be of limited long-term value to the medical practitioner. What, then is the correct use of a museum specimen?

WORKING WITH MUSEUM SPECIMENS

A skill that is of great value to the medical practitioner is the ability to observe, to see what is before one's eyes. This is much harder than it sounds, since even if we are willing to place some effort into looking, our perception is often distorted by preconception. Assuming that observation has been made with care and accuracy, the next task is to describe what has been seen. Simple and concise descriptions should be used. A good description is one which can be understood and visualised by someone reading or hearing it (an exercise in communication that is well worth attempting). To achieve a meaningful description the observer must be able to recognise and describe normal anatomy. This will form a point of reference for a comparative description of diseased tissue.

After the abnormalities have been recognised and described, it is necessary to suggest the basis of the changes in terms of general pathological mechanisms operating at the cell and tissue level. This is not the same as a full diagnosis. For example, abnormal pallor in a tissue might be fully explained by an infiltration of white blood cells. This could in turn have an inflammatory or a neoplastic basis. More detailed diagnosis beyond inflammatory or neoplastic may only be possible with the benefit of prior knowledge or histological examination. However, a differential diagnosis (in order of likelihood) can be offered. A single specimen may contain two or more pathological lesions which will often be related causally, and appropriate mechanisms may be suggested. Finally comes the correlation with clinical symptoms and signs.

In summary, the steps in studying the museum specimen are:

1. Observe, distinguishing normal from abnormal
2. Describe the changes using clear and succinct language
3. Reason or hypothesise (regarding underlying mechanisms)
4. Provide a differential diagnosis
5. Link two or more separate lesions within a stepwise or pathogenetic sequence
6. Correlate with clinical symptoms and signs

THE SUFFIXES –OSIS AND –ITIS

The Greeks added –osis to words to create a noun out of a verb denoting an action or process. Most disease terms ending in –osis are non-inflammatory and often generalised processes, whereas –itis indicates an inflammatory mechanism. There are exceptions. The tubercles or granulomas of tuberculosis were once thought to be tumours and not inflammatory lesions. We also have aspergillosis and brucellosis. Conversely, diffuse or leather-bottle gastric cancer was thought to be an inflammatory process by early microscopists, hence the term linitis plastica.

LINKING APPEARANCES WITH MECHANISMS

The link between appearances and underlying mechanisms can rarely be made intuitively or without prior knowledge. Autopsies were performed for centuries without shedding much light on disease mechanisms until the second half of the nineteenth century and the advent of microscopy. Now, in retrospect, one can make several generalisations about the gross structure of disease and what this is likely to imply in terms of mechanisms.

The description of a disease begins with the affected organ. Organs are composed of multiple tissues arranged in layers, linings or coverings and traversed by structures such as ducts, vessels or nerves. Observation must be applied systematically to each tissue or structure contributing to an organ. Solid organs are generally mounted to reveal a sectioned parenchymal surface, while hollow organs are opened to reveal the mucosal lining (as in the case of the gut, for example). An organ is rarely destroyed entirely by the pathological process. An exception is a small organ such as the ovary which may become completely replaced by a bulky tumour. A solid organ may be increased or reduced in size (it may not be possible to recognise this in a single slice) but generally retains its usual shape. A small organ may have atrophied with age or be from a neonate or child. Certain normal structures or tissues may cause confusion. The yellow or orange fat in the hilum of the kidney or spleen or the papillary choroid plexus in the ventricles of the brain may be incorrectly construed as pathological. Sectioned lymph nodes in the gut mesentery are often not recognised for what they are, even when brought to a student's attention.

FOCAL, MULTIFOCAL AND DIFFUSE DISEASE

In the case of solid organs such as the liver, kidney, thyroid gland or spleen, it is useful to classify disease appearances as: (1) focal (solitary), (2) multifocal or (3) diffuse. Multifocality means that several discrete lesions are separated by normal parenchyma whereas no entirely normal parenchyma is seen in a diffuse process. Examples of diffuse processes are provided in the end stage diseases (see Chapter 33), hyperplasia and hypertrophy (page 105), lobar pneumonia (page 77), congestion (page 113) and polycystic disease of kidney. Many diffuse patterns are caused by cells or cellular products spreading or infiltrating the interstitial spaces between parenchymal cells. White blood cells are adapted for such a mode of spread and will do so on a massive scale in haematological malignancies. Amyloidosis (page 92) is an example of diffuse deposition of a proteinaceous material derived from various types of protein precursor. With the notable exceptions of leukaemia, lymphoma and diffuse type gastric cancer, neoplasms are generally either focal (primary) or multifocal (secondary). Splenic lymphoma may selectively replace the white pulp to produce a multifocal pattern.

Inflammatory processes (acute or chronic) may be focal, multifocal or diffuse. Examples of discrete lesions are the solitary abscess and tuberculoma. Multifocal inflammatory processes include multiple abscesses, bronchopneumonia, bronchiolitis, and miliary tuberculosis. Given the generalised vascular response and infiltrative ability of neutrophils, acute inflammation is by and large a diffuse process, although may be localised to an anatomical region (such as the appendix or subarachnoid space). In inflamed tissues that include a serous membrane, for example peritoneum, pleura or pericardium, involvement of the latter (serositis) presents as an adherent shaggy fibrinous exudate. Infarcts may be focal or multifocal and are typically wedge-shaped and well demarcated from surrounding tissues.

COLOUR

Colour is a useful guide to disease processes, but students often incorrectly interpret dark tissue as diseased and pale tissue as normal. The majority of pathological processes in pots are pale (pale infarcts of kidney, spleen and heart, tumours, tumour necrosis, granulomas and lobar pneumonia). The expectation that disease should be dark may be related to archetypal images of blackened digits affected by frost-bite, the desiccated and mummified digits result-ing from ischaemia or the blackened tissues associated with gas gangrene. Dark tissue in museum specimens that is diffuse is likely to be normal (venous infarction of the gut and pseudomelanosis coli would be notable exceptions). A thin red line representing hyperaemic granulation tissue is seen at the edge of pale infarcts that are several days old. The granula-tion tissue (pyogenic membrane) lining an abscess cavity forms a thin red line which is coated with an equally thin layer of pale, cream-coloured fibrin. The pus itself is often lost, leaving an empty cavity.

Massive haemorrhage, appearing as zones of dark tissue, is usually traumatic or second-ary to spontaneous rupture of an arterial aneurysm (see below). It is not usual to observe extensive haemorrhage within tumours. Exceptions include teratoma of the testis with choriocarcinomatous elements, renal cell carcinoma and malignant tumours of vascular ori-gin. The early pale infarct may be associated with haemorrhage in surrounding tissues. Infarcts of the lung and gut are dark red (when fresh). Brain infarcts often show secondary haemorrhage.

Tumour that is dark brown or black is likely to be malignant melanoma. Jet black deposits in the lung parenchyma and regional lymph nodes will be carbon derived from cigarette smoke or urban pollution. Preserved fatty tissue is relatively hard and opaque. Whilst it retains the yellow colour of its fresh state, it may darken or assume an orange tint. Intracellu-lar deposits of lipid, such as cholesterol within collections of macrophages, also appear yellow.

HOLES

Sections through solid organs may reveal 'holes'. Small holes may also be observed in the mucosal lining of hollow organs. Holes may be: (1) cysts, (2) cystic degeneration consequent to necrosis in infarcts or tumours, (3) abscess cavities, (4) the necrotic centres of granulomas, (5) air filled sacs or cavities, or (6) dilated (ectatic) tubes cut transversely.

A cyst is a collection of fluid or semi-solid material that is enclosed within a sac with an epithelial lining. Cysts are formed on the basis of simple obstruction of an otherwise normal gland or tubule, as a complication of tissue maldevelopment, in the course of neoplastic change or in the context of parasitic invasion (e.g. hydatid disease). The contents of cysts will vary according to the type of underlying epithelium: keratin in the case of epidermal or pilar (sebaceous) cysts, protein-rich fluid in the case of either simple or neoplastic cysts lined by a serous epithelium, mucin in the case of neoplastic cysts lined by mucinous epithelium, and sebaceous material in benign ovarian teratomas (dermoid cysts). The more fluid contents will be lost within museum preparations but mucin may persist as transparent, semi-opaque or opaque glairy material.

Cystic spaces form as a result of necrosis followed by liquefaction, as in the case of cerebral infarction or abscess formation. Cavities within tumours may arise following ischaemic necrosis or when haemorrhage is followed by lysis and absorption of the blood clot. The pale caseous (cheesy) material within tuberculous granulomas may disappear leaving a space. Air-filled cavities occur in the lungs in a broad range of pulmonary diseases causing damage at all levels of the bronchial tree. For example, cavities complicating tuberculosis occur following granulomatous destruction of an airway. Dilated and ulcerated (bronchiectatic) bronchi resemble abscess cavities when sectioned transversely. Destruction of alveolar walls in emphysema results in dilatation of the distal airways to form holes or bullae (sacs).

POUCHES AND BULGES

Outpouching or bulging may affect hollow tubes and may be developmental or acquired. Acquired outpouching or localised dilatation requires a pressure gradient across the wall and a weakness of the wall itself. The weakness may be the result of a destructive process or a normal anatomical defect. Localised dilatations within the cardiovascular system are called aneurysms (page 124). Arterial walls may be weakened by atherosclerosis, infection or immune complex deposition, whereas the left ventricular wall is weakened by ischaemic necrosis. Mucosal outpouchings in the gastrointestinal tract are called diverticula. These occur most commonly in the sigmoid colon and herniate outwards along the paths of penetrating vessels.

SHAPES AND CONTOURS OF NEOPLASMS

Benign neoplasms and relatively non-aggressive early cancers originating in epithelial surfaces usually grow upwards and outwards as an exophytic or polypoid growth. They may be relatively solid with a lobulated surface or composed of delicate fronds, finger-like villi or leaves covered by epithelium (Fig. 3).

Viewed from their epithelial aspect, many advanced carcinomas present as an ulcer with a raised, rolled, everted edge. The cut surface of a primary cancer appears as a mass of white tissue with an irregular border that infiltrates and destroys the adjacent structures. By contrast, metastatic deposits are characterised not only by their multiplicity but also (when located with the parenchyma of solid organs) by their perfectly spherical nature. Adenocarcinomas secreting abundant mucus show a sponge-like or honeycomb appearance on section. This appearance is explained by the accumulation of mucin within distended glands. Cancers are generally solid, but benign and malignant neoplasms of the ovary, teratomas of the testis and some pancreatic cancers are cystic.

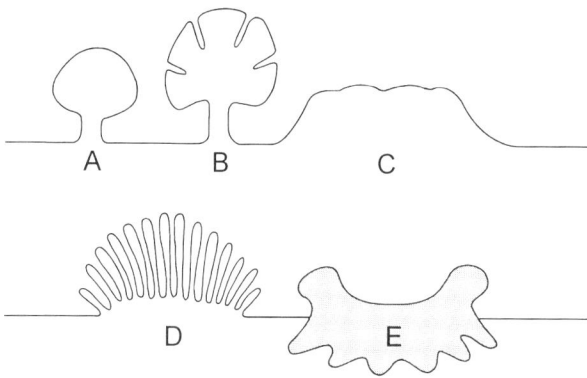

Figure 3 Contours of neoplasms: pedunculated polyp (A), pedunculated polyp with lobulated surface (B), sessile polyp (C), sessile polyp with villous architecture (D), ulcerated cancer with raised, rolled, everted edge (E).

MICROSCOPIC EXAMINATION

For the uninitiated, the microscopic image is a bewildering kaleidoscope of colours and patterns. The main colours in a haematoxylin and eosin stained section are blue (nuclei), pink (cytoplasm) and intensely eosinophilic or orange (red blood cells). Because normal nuclei are relatively small, most normal tissues are pink. This can be appreciated when stained sections are viewed with the naked eye against a white background. Inflammatory cells, notably lymphocytes, have densely stained nuclei and little cytoplasm. Some normal tissues, princi-pally lymph nodes, are lymphocyte rich and stain blue. Certain diseases impart a blue colour to tissues. Disorders associated with a heavy inflammatory cell infiltrate and neoplasms composed of cells with increased nuclear–cytoplasmic ratios are the main examples. Con-versely, necrotic tissues lack nuclei and appear pinker than normal.

The beginner needs a reasonable knowledge of normal histology and must also be familiar with microscopic appearances at low, medium and high magnification. It is worth examining gross specimens with a hand lens and comparing the appearances to low-power histology. With a little practice, most tissues can be readily diagnosed by holding the histological section up to a light. Tissues that are often confused by students are prostate versus breast (only the latter includes fat) and the regions of the gut (only small bowel has villi).

The microscopic study of disease provides opportunities for developing observational and descriptive skills and a deepening understanding of the underlying mechanisms of dis-ease. The medical student is not expected to make a tissue diagnosis or develop pattern recognition skills. Far more important in the long term is the ability to understand, explain and act on a report from an anatomical pathologist. The salient microscopic features of the major disease categories are described throughout this book.

— PART II —

INJURY, INFLAMMATION AND IMMUNITY

10

INFLAMMATION:
HISTORICAL PERSPECTIVES

Nothing is more satisfying for the mind than to be able to follow
a discovery from its very origin up to its latest developments

Louis Pasteur

What is infection?

The four cardinal signs of inflammation, documented by the Roman writer Aulus Celsus in the first century AD, describe the classical appearances of acute inflammation as observed in the skin and subjacent structures. Rubor, tumor, calor and dolor equate with redness, swelling, heat and pain respectively, and serve as a potent reminder of the critical involvement of the microvasculature in the acute inflammatory process. Marcello Malpighi (1628–1694), professor of anatomy at Bologna, was the first to observe and describe the microscopic capillary network with the aid of live frog preparations. The London-based Scottish anatomist and surgeon John Hunter (1728–1793) treated and studied gunshot wounds and perceived inflammation as a ubiquitous and beneficial process manifested not only by the features described by Celsus, but also by the discharge of 'laudable pus'. Giovanni Battista Morgagni (1682–1771), the Paduan professor of anatomy who was the first to develop clinicopathological correlation through systematic autopsy examination, described the curious process whereby the lung is transmuted to liver (red hepatisation), now known to be an early stage in the evolution of classical lobar pneumonia caused by *Streptococcus pneumoniae*.

Xavier Bichat (1771–1802) and his colleagues in the University of Paris extended Hunter's observations by describing the universal appearance of acute inflammation within internal structures such as the serous membranes covering the heart, lung and abdominal organs and the mucous membrane of the gut. Julius Cohnheim (1839–1884) took the observations of Malpighi a step further by inducing inflammation and documenting the vascular changes in semitransparent live frog tissues. In 1927 Thomas Lewis introduced the concept that chemical mediators (histamine) brought about the vascular changes associated with inflammation. However, while it was now abundantly clear that inflammation is a response to injury such as trauma or chemical irritation and not a disease in itself, discovery of the principal pathogen, the micro-organism, came first through the pioneering contribution of the French chemist

Louis Pasteur (1822–1895) and subsequently with the identification of the causative agents of anthrax and tuberculosis by the German microbiologist Robert Koch (1843–1910) (Maulitz, 1993).

GERMS AND CONTAGION

The concept that certain diseases were contagious predated the work of Pasteur by centuries, but the agents of contagion were constructs of a highly theoretical nature. The ancient Greeks were aware that diseases such as tuberculosis and scabies were transmissible, but blamed such factors as exhaled putrid air. The Hippocratic Corpus focuses on combinations of 'airs, waters and places' as the explanation for disease outbreaks. Blame was placed upon 'miasma' or putrid air derived from stagnant marshes, corpses, sick persons, excreta, vapours emanating through rocky clefts from the bowels of the earth and so on (Hannaway, 1993). This concept of disease was accepted through the centuries to the time of Pasteur, serving as the most reasonable alternative to divine punishment. The modern equivalents of the concept of miasma might be greenhouse gases, natural and artificial pollutants and cigarette smoke. The normally pragmatic Galen (130–201 AD) mused on the concept of 'bad seeds' in the putrid air and suggested that they might be inhaled and lie dormant until activated by some stimulus. This was an attempt to explain both contagion and the variable susceptibility of individuals to disease. The 'bad seeds' were not considered to be microbes but invisible atom-like particles (concepts dating back to Democritus 460–370 BC and Anaxagoras (500–428 BC) (Jackson, 1988).

Girolamo Fracastoro (1478–1553) reflected on the infective nature of syphilis, a disease that derives its name from the hero of his poem. Credited with the introduction of a germ theory of disease, Fracastoro believed that 'fomites' (such as articles of clothing) could carry contagion. However, it is probable that he regarded his 'seeds' of disease as non-living particles, similar to those of Galen.

Paracelsus (1493–1541) saw disease as affecting the body from without. Furthermore, in contrast with the prevailing humoral theory, he believed that the body was affected locally and not as a whole. The views of this influential mystic are certainly in accord with the behaviour of many infective illnesses.

In the seventeenth century the microscopic 'animalcules' of Antony van Leeuwenhoek (1632–1723) provoked lively speculation about their role in nature and mode of reproduction. However, no connection between microscopic animals and disease was made. By the eighteenth century some diseases, such as smallpox, were understood to be highly infectious, whereas others, such as malaria, were not passed directly from person to person but occurred in certain localities. These diseases were grouped together as fevers involving the ripening (coction) of morbid (peccant) matter within the body. If this matter was successfully expelled through the body's pores or orifices (similar to the laudable pus of Hunter) the crisis was resolved and the patient recovered. This was Thomas Sydenham's (1624–1689) 'Hippocratic' view of disease. Sydenham, regarded as the founder of modern clinical medicine, believed that disease processes had a natural life of their own and that the patient was helped by as little interference as possible by the physician.

By the mid-nineteenth century, bacteria had been described by microscopists, and terms such as bacillus, vibrio, bacterium and spirochaete were introduced prior to the work of Pasteur. However, diseases that are now known to be caused by infective agents were still classified as being either contagious or due to miasma, or to a problematical combination of the two (Pelling, 1993). Pasteur's great idea was to separate the chemistry of non-living nature from that of living nature, but he found a grey area when he studied wine production. Once he concluded that the fermentation of wine was dependent on the presence of bacteria, the analogy could be drawn with the ripening, coction and fermentation associated with disease processes (these terms had been in use for centuries). He also pointed out that just as certain bacteria were associated with a particular type of fermentation, so could specific bacterial agents be linked with particular diseases. He went on to apply the same principle to putrefaction. With the advent of the cell theory, ideas about the spontaneous generation of organised structures from decaying matter were beginning to emerge. The concept of the spontaneous generation of life was perceived by many as irreligious. Therefore Pasteur's experiments had great popular appeal because the process of fermentation (which evoked the idea of growth) was shown to require the presence of a preexisting life form.

Whilst many infective diseases involved decay and pustulation, tuberculosis with its tumour-like tubercles was perceived as being more like cancer. This concept as much as the importance of the disease itself would have made Koch's discovery of the causative acid fast bacillus (*Mycobacterium tuberculosis*) all the more remarkable at the time. Koch postulated that a micro-organism could be shown to be the cause of a disease if it was isolated from diseased tissue, grown artificially in culture, transmitted to another individual and produced the same disease. This model sparked a bacteriological revolution in Germany, whereas Pasteur and his followers focused their attention on developing the principles of vaccination.

IMPACT OF AN INFECTIVE THEORY OF DISEASE

The infective theory of disease, with its emphasis on a specific foreign organism entering the body and causing a localised disease (an ontological concept beginning with a preexisting external cause that results in an internal effect), provided the single greatest challenge to the ancient holistic and humoralistic view of disease that stressed the individuality of the whole person (it is often incorrectly thought that holistic medicine is a new concept). In the infective model, a formerly healthy individual becomes the anonymous victim of an aggressive pathogen, and may be cured by the killing of the causative agent. Paul Ehrlich's (1854–1915) dream of 'magic bullets' became a reality following Alexander Fleming's (1881–1955) discovery of a naturally occurring antibiotic substance within the mould *Penicillium notatum* which acted specifically upon bacteria.

The success achieved by the use of antibiotics in reducing morbidity and mortality due to infective disease, coupled with the perception of the growing scourge of cardiovascular disease, cancer and 'degenerative' disease associated with ageing has rekindled the much older belief in the role of non-living environmental agents. However, today's miasma would include toxic chemicals, air pollutants, radiation and so on. This resurgence of ancient beliefs has been coupled with a renewed focus on holistic medicine, including the need to balance the health of body, mind and soul.

Nevertheless, humankind has been reminded of the lurking danger of the microbe following the discovery of AIDS and its causative human immunodeficiency virus (HIV), the relatively recent realisation that chronic gastritis has a bacterial cause (*Helicobacter pylori*), the growing menace of bacterial resistance to antibiotics, the resurgence of tuberculosis and venereal disease amongst the world's growing poor and disadvantaged, and the appreciation that many cancers and possibly even arterial disease are caused by infective agents. The microbe has not become part of history but will continue to shape human destiny by impacting upon the lives of millions. Furthermore it is inevitable that specific micro-organisms will be shown to be the initiating agents of many chronic diseases for which the causes are presently unknown.

DEFENCE MECHANISMS

Once the reaction known as inflammation was shown to be a defensive response to invasion of the body by pathogenic micro-organisms, researchers began to uncover the underlying mechanisms involved. Two great ideas were to emerge before the end of the nineteenth century—the concepts of cellular and serum factor (humoral) defence systems. Russian zoologist Elie Metchnikoff (1845–1916) decided to study aquatic invertebrates while holidaying with his family in Sicily. He observed motile cells within starfish larvae and conducted experiments to determine whether these phagocytes (meaning cells that eat) had a defensive role against micro-organisms. His initial positive results were published in 1884.

In 1890 Behring and Kitasato demonstrated the presence in serum of an antitoxin to the lethal toxins produced by diphtheria and tetanus. The German microbiologist Paul Ehrlich (1854–1915) introduced the term antibody (antikörper) in 1891, and went on to characterise the chemical nature of the interactions between toxins and antibodies. The cellular and antibody theories were initially deemed to be incompatible. It was thought that one or the other system should be enough. Robert Koch sided with the antibody theory. Eventually both theories were accepted as correct and complementary and Metchnikoff (instated at the Pasteur Institute) and Ehrlich were joint Nobel prize winners in 1908 (Weindling, 1993).

The quest for vaccines and antitoxins provided the main impetus for the development of what Medawar (1974) has described as 'old immunology'. The old immunology began when the English physician Edward Jenner (1749–1823) decided to put the 'old wives' tale' regarding the protective benefit of cowpox against subsequent exposure to smallpox to the test. Pasteur commemorated Jenner's pioneering achievement by introducing the term vaccination (*vacca* and *vache* mean cow in Latin and French respectively) and his Paris Institute paved the way for key developments in this field.

The concepts of old and new immunology will be developed in Chapter 14, emphasising mainly the underlying mechanisms as well as their morphological counterparts regarded as having diagnostic importance.

REFERENCES

Hannaway, C. (1993) Environment and miasmata. In *Companion Encyclopedia of the History of Medicine*, volume 1, edited by W.F. Bynum and R. Porter. London and New York: Routledge, pp 292–308.

Jackson, R. (1988) *Doctors and Diseases in the Roman Empire*. University of Oklahoma Press: Norman and London.

Maulitz, R.C. (1993) The pathological tradition. In *Companion Encyclopedia of the History of Medicine*, volume 1, edited by W.F. Bynum & R. Porter, pp. 169–191. London and New York: Routledge.

Medawar, P.B. (1974) The new immunology. *Hosp Pract*, **9**, 48.

Pelling, M. (1993) Contagion, germ theory, specificity. In *Companion Encyclopedia of the History of Medicine*, volume 1, edited by W.F. Bynum & R. Porter, pp. 309–334. London and New York: Routledge.

Weindling, P. (1993) The immunological tradition. In *Companion Encyclopedia of the History of Medicine*, volume 1, edited by W.F. Bynum & R. Porter, pp. 192–204. London and New York: Routledge.

11

THE INJURED CELL

What is your substance, whereof are you made?

William Shakespeare

When does a cell die?

CELL STRUCTURE AND FUNCTION

Virchow's belief in the cell as the unit of life and seat of disease has stood the test of time and continues to drive modern biomedical research. A key development in the consolidation of the cell theory of disease was the construction of the prototype electron microscope by Ruska in Germany in 1933. This instrument allowed the fine detail of the cell to be resolved by the scatter pattern of an electron beam passing through an ultrathin section. However, the technology for preparing and staining sections that would allow the structures shown in Figure 4 to be resolved was slow to develop. The crucial link between the structure and function of the cytoplasmic 'organelles' was demonstrated by the work of Claude, Palade and deDuve. They used ultracentrifugation to separate the organelles, characterised the purified subfractions biochemically and finally correlated function with structure by submitting the purified fractions for electron microscopic study. Their efforts were rewarded by shared Nobel prizes in 1974. Functions of cell structures, particularly those that relate to an under-standing of cell injury, are summarised in the following sections.

The cell membrane

The cell membrane is not merely a membranous bag housing the cytoplasm and nucleus, but serves as a semipermeable membrane capable of maintaining large chemical gradients between the intracellular and extracellular compartments. Additionally the cell membrane is studded with receptors and molecules involved in adhesion and communication (see page 104).

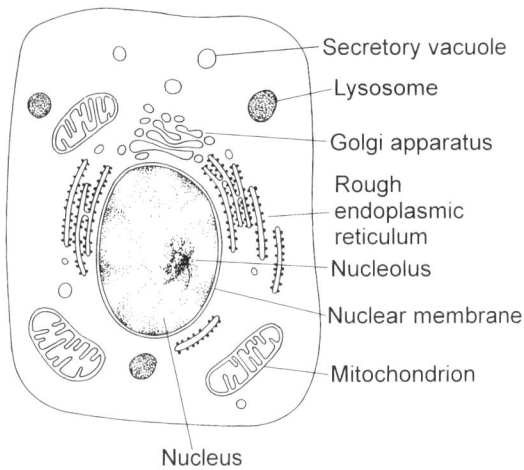

Figure 4 Schematic diagram of the ultrastructural appearances of a generic cell

Mitochondria

Mitochondria generate the energy requirements of the cell. They are the seat of aerobic respiration, in which cytochrome oxidase catalyses the four-electron reduction of O_2 to H_2O, a process leading to the generation of high-energy ATP (adenosine triphosphate).

Lysosomes

These membrane bound structures contain hydrolases such as proteases (e.g. cathepsin G), lipases and glucosidases. They are very numerous in phagocytic cells, neutrophils and macrophages. Phagocytosed bacteria are digested when the phagosome fuses with lysosomes to form a phagolysosome.

Endoplasmic reticulum

Smooth endoplasmic reticulum is the site of lipid and steroid synthesis, whereas protein is synthesised in the rough endoplasmic reticulum studded with ribosomes (formed of ribosomal RNA). Post-translational modification of protein in the form of glycosylation (addition of carbohydrate) occurs in the Golgi apparatus. Secretory vacuoles bud off from the latter and pass to the cell membrane to be exported.

Nucleus

The nucleus is enclosed by a nuclear membrane and comprises chromosomes and a nucleolus. The material forming the chromosomes is called chromatin and consists of DNA and protein. The chromosomes only assume their characteristic condensed form during mitosis (cell division) (Fig. 5). During the remainder of the cell cycle (interphase), chromosomes are highly dispersed and cannot be seen individually. Chromatin exists either in a densely packed form (heterochromatin) or a more dispersed form (euchromatin). Euchromatin is the form that is being genetically expressed (transcribed). Chromatin has a very complicated structure. Short lengths of DNA (about 200 base pairs) are packaged up with proteins (histones) to form complexes known as nucleosomes. These are assembled as repeating units into higher order

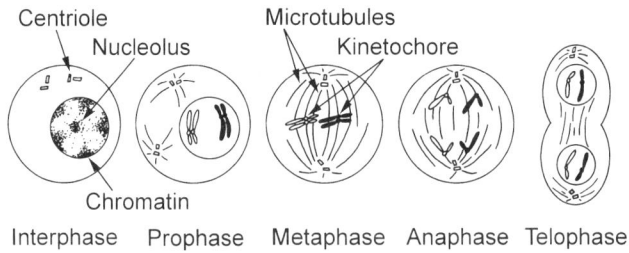

Figure 5 Mitotic cell division showing two duplicated chromosomes. During metaphase the chromosomes are attached to the spindle (formed of microtubules) by means of the kinetochore. The spindle contracts to draw the chromosomes apart during anaphase. Daughter cells are formed during telophase.

chromatin structures. The nucleolus is the site of ribosomal RNA synthesis and ribosome assembly.

CELL INJURY

Cell injury is classified as being either reversible or irreversible. There is no morphologically defined point that marks the passage of injury from reversible to irreversible. Cells may be injured by numerous agents: microbes, ischaemia (loss of blood supply), temperature extremes, chemicals, drugs, radiation or the immune system. The aim of therapy in the situation of the threatened cell is to remove or neutralise the injurious agent and prevent cells from reaching the point of no return: irreversible injury leading to cell death. Reversible cell injury is manifested histologically by hydropic swelling in which cells are enlarged and filled with a pale cytoplasm. The usual cause is a temporary failure of the sodium pump mechanism in the cell membrane. Sodium and water enter the cell and this accounts for the morphological change. As stated above, the influx of calcium ions into the cell marks the transition of reversible to irreversible injury. At the electron microscopic level there is distension of the endoplasmic reticulum and mitochondrial swelling.

NECROSIS

The term necrosis describes the morphological changes that follow the death of cells contained within a living organism. If the acute injury is sufficiently severe the cell will die. The most common cause of pathological cell death is ischaemia. Other causes include extreme temperatures and toxic chemicals. In most tissues this gives rise to a characteristic morphological change called coagulative necrosis. (This term was introduced by Cohnheim and Weigert, early followers of Virchow, who incorrectly believed that necrosis was precipitated by coagulation of fibrinogen.) Necrosis is distinguished from the autolysis seen postmortem when cells are digested by released lysosomal enzymes and there is no tissue response. Necrosis is also distinguished from active or programmed cell death known as apoptosis (page 102).

Histological examination of well-developed coagulative necrosis reveals the tissue structure in ghostly outline. The cell cytoplasm persists and is stained deeply with eosin. This is due partly to the rapid degradation of basophilic RNA and partly to an increased affinity for eosin. The nuclei disappear. Prior to their disappearance, the nuclei may be fragmented (karyorrhexis), shrunken and darkly staining (pyknosis) or may simply dissolve (karyolysis) (Fig. 6). Since necrosis is occurring in a living organism, there will be an inflammatory reaction culminating in the removal of the dead tissue by a process called organisation.

Liquefactive necrosis occurs when there is rapid dissolution of cells. This is the usual outcome of necrosis in the brain that is of ischaemic origin. Formation of an abscess may also be described as liquefactive necrosis. Fat necrosis affects adipose tissue and is a typical feature associated with acute inflammation of the pancreas (pancreatitis). The enzyme lipase released by the injured pancreas converts triglycerides into free fatty acids. These are in turn converted to calcium soaps which appear macroscopically as white chalky areas and histologically as amorphous blue deposits. The fourth type of necrosis is caseous necrosis, associated typically with tuberculosis. The necrotic tissue has a soft, dry and cheese-like consistency.

The molecular events leading to coagulative necrosis have been studied in detail in experimental (animal) models in which periods of ischaemia (of the heart, for example) can be accurately controlled. Loss of the ability of the cell membrane to maintain chemical gradients is the first critical step. The gradient is greatest for calcium ions which are highly active biologically. Cells that are rich in mitochondria and depend on aerobic respiration for the production of ATP are particularly sensitive to the effects of ischaemia. ATP is required for the maintenance of chemical gradients across membranes.

Failure of mitochondrial recovery upon restoration of the blood supply and re-oxygenation is the second critical hallmark of irreversible injury. Paradoxically, re-oxygenation may make matters worse, a phenomenon known as reperfusion injury (Gross ct al., 1986; Hearse et al., 1993). The injury occurs when oxygen is only partially reduced, giving rise to active oxygen species (superoxide, H_2O_2 and hydroxyl radicals). These are by-products of the enzyme xanthine oxidase acting upon purines derived from ATP catabolism. Production of reactive oxygen species by phagocytic cells also contributes to tissue damage. The killing of cells by ionising radiation and many toxic chemicals is also mediated by reactive oxygen species. Genetic damage is caused by the same mechanism and may lead to carcinogenesis. A third critical step in ischaemic necrosis is the degradation of phospholipids within cell membranes by phospholipases.

The extent of cell injury is limited by a diverse family of proteins called heat shock proteins or chaperonins (Knowlton, 1995). The primary function of these molecules is to assist in the

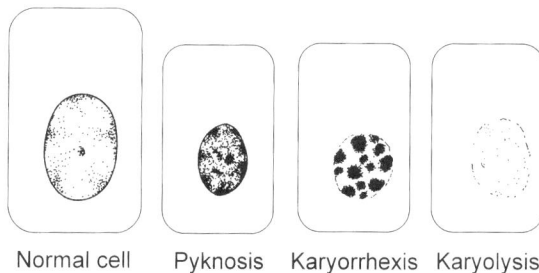

Normal cell   Pyknosis   Karyorrhexis   Karyolysis

Figure 6 Nuclear changes in the necrotic cell

folding and translocation of intracellular proteins. These molecules therefore rescue proteins that have become unfolded as a result of cell injury. A particular heat shock protein, ubiquitin, clears proteins that have been damaged beyond repair.

ABNORMAL CELL STORAGE

Lipid and carbohydrate

All cells are adapted for some degree of storage (such as that required for nutritional needs) and some are adapted for large scale storage (e.g. fat by adipocytes). Abnormal intracellular storage is seen in various pathological conditions, particularly in the liver. Triglycerides accumulate in liver cells damaged by alcohol or when the delivery of fatty acids is increased as in diabetes mellitus or starvation. Fat is lost during tissue processing but is visualised histologically by the presence of empty globules of varying size. Excessive storage of cytoplasmic glycogen is seen in diabetes and also in rare autosomal recessive conditions in which there is a deficiency of enzymes involved in glycogen breakdown. Failure to break down complex lipids and glycosaminoglycans may also be the result of an inherited enzyme defect. These enzymes normally reside in lysosomes and the undigested products accumulate in these organelles.

Iron and copper

Twenty-five percent of the body's iron is stored as ferritin and haemosiderin. Haemosiderin is a partially denatured form of ferritin that forms aggregates visible microscopically as brown granules. Haemosiderin is stored within cells of the mononuclear/macrophage lineage, for example the Kupffer cells of the liver. This is not injurious, but excessive iron deposition involving parenchymal cells is toxic. Iron overload may result from repeated blood transfusions or from the autosomal recessive condition haemochromatosis. The organs at principal risk are the liver, heart and pancreas. In Wilson's disease, also an autosomal recessive condition, copper accumulates in the liver and brain.

Lipofuscin

Lipofuscin is a golden brown 'wear and tear' pigment found in cells that are permanent (neurons and cardiac muscle) or stable (liver). This is a normal cell constituent and the amount increases with age. It is often more marked in organs showing atrophy. Lipofuscin is derived from partially degraded cell membranes and is contained within autophagic vacuoles.

Melanin

Melanin is the dark brown or black pigment produced by the melanocytes of the skin and passed into adjacent epithelial cells. Melanin absorbs ultraviolet light and therefore protects the skin from damage. The amount of melanin produced by organelles called melanosomes is responsible for skin colour. Inflammatory skin lesions resulting in apoptosis are marked by the presence of melanophages (macrophages that have engulfed apoptotic bodies containing melanin). Regression of malignant melanoma is also associated with the presence of melanophages. 'Melanosis coli' in which the colonic musosal lining accumulates brown pigment is a misnomer. The pigment is related to lipfuscin and the condition results from chronic injury to the epithelium of the large bowel caused by purgative abuse.

Carbon

Carbon is a jet black pigment visualised in the alveolar macrophages and lymphatic system of the lung. The hilar and mediastinal lymph nodes of coal miners and smokers and even urban dwellers may be perfectly black, but on its own carbon is inert and harmless.

CALCIFICATION

There are two types of calcification: dystrophic and metastatic. Dystrophic calcification occurs in areas of necrosis or in diseased and relatively inert tissues in which there has been extensive fibrosis. Relatively common disorders associated with calcification include tuberculosis, atherosclerosis, and heart valvular disease. Certain neoplasms, particularly those with a papillary architecture, show calcification. The tips of the finger-like papillae are prone to ischaemic necrosis with secondary calcification. Calcifying cancers include papillary carcinoma of thyroid, papillary ovarian neoplasms, and the central nervous system tumours meningioma and oligodendroglioma. Histologically, calcium salts (mainly phosphate) appear as amorphous, granular basophilic material or as crystalline deposits. The calcified bodies in cancers are often quite large and show concentric lamellae. They are called psammoma bodies.

Metastatic calcification occurs in normal tissues in subjects with hypercalcaemia. Common causes of hypercalcaemia include overproduction of parathyroid hormone (for example by a parathyroid adenoma), vitamin D intoxication and excessive consumption of alkali. Metastatic calcification is most common in sites of ion exchange: alveoli of lung, gastric mucosa and renal tubules.

Most stones formed in the gallbladder, urinary system or salivary gland ducts contain calcium salts, though some gallbladder stones may be composed exclusively of cholesterol or of bile pigment. Hypercalcaemia is a cause of renal stones, but stone formation is also aggravated by local factors such as stasis and infection.

AGEING OF CELLS

This is a large and important subject, but there is still no explanation for ageing. Whilst environmental factors such as exposure to ultraviolet light and smoking accelerate the ageing process (particularly noticeable in the skin), ageing itself is likely to be endogenous and under genetic control.

Ageing has been studied at the level of the cell, and studies have shown that normal fibroblasts have a limited lifespan in culture. Fibroblasts from subjects with a rare disorder called progeria who suffer from premature ageing have a reduced lifespan under the same cell culture conditions. By contrast, malignant cells may be immortalised.

One mechanism for genetically programmed ageing may be gradual telomere reduction during cell division (Harley & Villeponteau, 1995). Telomeres stabilise the terminal portions of chromosomes and anchor them to the nuclear matrix. Telomeres shorten spontaneously with each cell division, but may be reconstituted with the enzyme telomerase. It has been suggested that telomerase upregulation could account for the immortality of cancer cells. However, cells lacking telomerase activity can undergo oncogenic transformation and produce tumours in nude mice (Blasco et al., 1997).

SUMMARY

This chapter has focused on the cellular response to injury in terms of recovery, death or the abnormal accumulation of metabolic products. Another option is considered in Chapter 16, namely adaptation.

REFERENCES

Blasco, M.A., Lee, H.W., Hande, M.P., Samper, E., Landsdorp, P.M., DePinho, R. & Greider, C.W. (1997) Telomere shortening and tumor formation by mouse cells lacking telomerase RNA. *Cell,* **91**, 25–34.

Gross, G.J., Farber, N.E., Hardman, H.F. & Warltier, D.C. (1986) Beneficial actions of superoxide dismutase and catalase in stunned myocardium of dogs. *Am J Physiol*, **250**, H372–377.

Harley, C.B. & Villeponteau, B. (1995) Telomeres and telomerase in aging and cancer. *Curr Opin Genet Dev,* **5**, 249–255.

Hearse, D.J., Maxwell, L., Saldanha, C. & Gavin, J.B. (1993) The myocardial vasculature during ischaemia and reperfusion: a target for injury and protection. *J Mol Cell Cardiol,* **25**, 759–800.

Knowlton, A.A. (1995) The role of heat shock proteins in the heart. *J Mol Cell Cardiol,* **27**, 121–131.

— 12 —

DEFENCES AGAINST INFECTION

The small is easily scattered

Tao Te Ching

How do bacteria provoke an inflammatory response?

KEEPING INFECTION AT BAY

In this book it has been a general policy to give an overview of the nature and appearances of the major disease processes, followed by some insight into the underlying mechanisms involved. As explained in Chapter 10, inflammation and the extrusion of 'corrupt matter' (pus) have long been viewed as a response to disease and not as a disease *per se*. This perception predated the discovery of infective micro-organisms. It is still a traditional policy for text-books of pathology to describe the mechanisms underlying the process of inflammation in considerable detail. The problem with this approach is that the mechanisms are complex, difficult to remember and of limited practical relevance in terms of both diagnosis and treat-ment. In general one does not treat the inflammation itself but the cause. Inflammation is a response by the tissues of the body to many injurious agents, but the most important are micro-organisms. The discovery of antibiotics means that few people in the Western world die prematurely of an infective illness. However, humankind as a species has survived for millennia without the benefit of either antibiotics or an understanding of the nature and life cycle of microbial agents. It is therefore necessary to ask why we do not succumb to the numerous infective organisms that daily threaten our existence. A very important clue that has helped us to answer this question is provided by the recognition of those unfortunate individuals who lack a specific component of the body's defence system.

PHYSICAL AND CHEMICAL BARRIERS TO INFECTION

The effectiveness of the skin in excluding pathogenic micro-organisms is demonstrated by the rapidity with which bacteria can enter the body through breaches in the skin, whether these be traumatic or surgical. As well as providing a physical barrier, sweat glands and sebaceous glands secrete lactic acid and fatty acids with bacteriocidal properties. The conjunctival membrane of the eye is far less robust than skin, but is bathed continuously with tears containing the enzyme lysozyme. As suggested by the name (and by its former name muramidase), this enzyme lyses bacterial cell walls. The same enzyme is found in phagocytic cells where it serves a similar role. The upper gastrointestinal tract is protected by a mucous barrier as well as by lysozyme. In addition the stomach is rendered sterile (with respect to the majority of micro-organisms) by its secretion of hydrochloric acid. The respiratory tract is protected by a barrier of mucus and the wave-like action of cilia (found at the apices of the specialised columnar epithelial cells) which waft particulate matter upwards. The colon contains a large population of bacteria. Not only are these useful commensals, for example assisting in the fermentation of plant fibre, but their presence protects the colon from parasitic invasion by pathogenic bacteria. The regular and complete emptying of such organs as the gallbladder and urinary bladder is of great importance in the maintenance of sterility.

CELLULAR AND HUMORAL FACTORS

The involvement of cellular and humoral factors in the defence against infection was appreciated by the end of the nineteenth century (see Chapter 10). The principal cell types involved in defence are shown in Figure 7. It is customary to divide inflammation into acute and chronic, a concept that will be developed in Chapter 13. Acute inflammation lasts only for a matter of days, whereas chronic inflammation continues for months, years or even a lifetime.

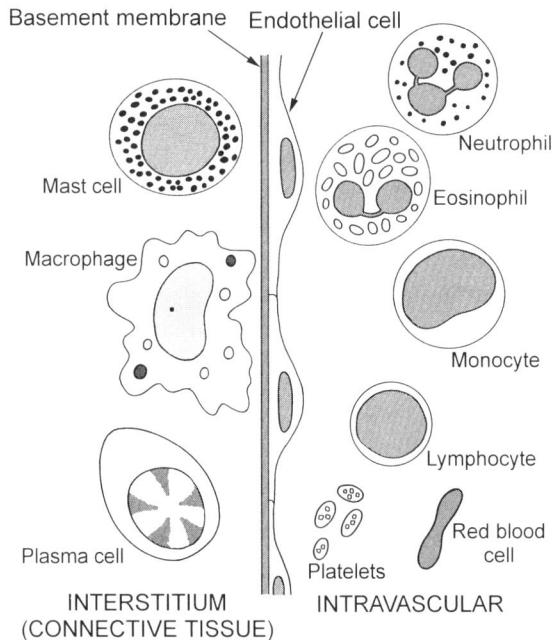

Figure 7 Inflammatory cell types shown within the compartments (intravascular and extravascular) where they are seen most typically in tissue sections

Both the type of infective micro-organism and the nature of the host's response determine the length of the inflammatory reaction. The cell type that plays the most critical role in acute inflammation is the neutrophil (polymorphonuclear leukocyte), whereas lymphocytes and cells of the mononuclear/macrophage lineage are the main participants in chronic inflammation. Neutrophils and macrophages are phagocytic (they literally eat invading organisms) whereas the remaining cells kill by releasing chemicals. The principal humoral factors are antibodies and a system of plasma proteins collectively known as complement. The existence of both was appreciated by the end of the nineteenth century. Complement and antibodies were distinguished by the fact that complement was heat labile (at 56 °C) whereas antibodies were not (Lachmann, 1992).

Immunity to infection may be classified as either natural or specific. Cellular and humoral factors operate in both natural and specific immunity. Neutrophils, eosinophils and macrophages (in simple phagocytic mode) are the cellular defences contributing to natural immunity and are supported by humoral factors in the form of complement. Although antibodies are secreted by terminally differentiated B lymphocytes (plasma cells) and are therefore considered under specific immunity (Chapter 14), they facilitate natural immunity by coating (opsonising) bacteria and thereby enhancing the effectiveness of phagocytic neutrophils.

NEUTROPHILS

These cells provide a major component of the defence against infection by micro-organisms. This is illustrated when a critical neutrophil function is deficient (as a result of an inherited deficiency). Affected individuals develop bacterial infections that are normally associated with the formation of pus. Examples of such pyogenic bacteria are staphyloccoci, streptococci, *E. coli* and *Klebsiella*. Additionally, these subjects will be at risk of fungal infections (such as *Candida albicans* and *Aspergillus*).

Neutrophils are generated within the bone marrow from myeloid precursors that give rise to other members of the granulocyte family (eosinophils and basophils). Once they enter the circulation, the half-life of neutrophils is a matter of hours. During pyogenic infections, the number of neutrophils rises sharply. Some of these will have been sequestered within the microvasculature of organs such as the spleen. Others will be maturing neutrophils that are released early from the marrow (recognised by their paucity of nuclear lobes). Neutrophils have a multilobated nucleus and finely granular cytoplasm. The granules are lysosomes containing a variety of enzymes including myeloperoxidase, lysozyme and cathepsin. The cell membrane has receptors for: (1) inflammatory mediators (e.g. components of complement such as C5a and platelet activating factor), (2) opsonised bacteria bearing the Fc portion of antibodies or the cleaved complement fragment C3b, and (3) adhesion molecules expressed by endothelial cells (the leukocyte integrin LFA-1 binds to intercellular adhesion molecule-1 (ICAM-1), while leukocyte receptors bearing the sialylated blood group Lewis X (SLe^x) bind to endothelial cell-leukocyte adhesion molecule–1 (ELAM-1) or E-selectin).

How is the neutrophil driven into a state of activity when its receptor encounters a ligand in the form of an inflammatory mediator? Briefly, the cytoplasmic domain becomes coupled with a regulatory G protein, critical in many such signalling pathways (page 100), and this activates phospholipase C in the neutrophil cell membrane. This in turn hydrolyses phosphatidylinositol biphosphate (PIP$_2$) to generate two highly reactive metabolites: diacylglycerol and inositol triphosphate (ITP). ITP causes release of stored intracellular Ca^{2+}, which triggers multiple events: (1) potentiation of phospholipase A_2 (which initiates synthesis of eicosanoids—see below), (2) activation of protein kinase C (which activates multiple proteins by phosphorylation), and (3) assembly of cytoskeletal elements involved in intracellular transport, movement and phagocytosis. Diacylglycerol also activates protein kinase C and is the precursor of arachidonic acid (see below).

The activated neutrophil performs a variety of complex functions mediated through its specialised receptors. An early step in the acute inflammatory process is neutrophil margination and rolling along the endothelial lining of the microvasculature. This is facilitated by the adhesion molecules noted above. Delivery of neutrophils in large numbers to an infected site is facilitated by histamine-induced dilatation of arterioles, which greatly increases the flow through the capillary bed. Additionally (in response to inflammatory mediators), the tight junctions of endothelial cells in the post-capillary venules open up, thus providing an exit route for activated neutrophils. Neutrophils are attracted to the site of infection by chemicals called chemotaxins and develop the capacity for independent amoeboid movement.

Phagocytosis requires the recognition of an opsonised bacterium, adherence of the bacterium to membrane receptors, invagination of the membrane around the bacterium, formation of a phagosome and fusion of the phagosome with neutrophil granules (lysosomes) to form a phagolysosome (Fig. 8). Phagocytosis is accompanied by a burst of metabolic activity. This culminates in the production of reactive oxygen species which serve as a further component of the neutrophil's bacteriocidal armamentarium. Dead and dying neutrophils are either extruded as pus or phagocytosed by macrophages (Savill et al., 1989).

NEUTROPHIL FAILURE

Failure to kill micro-organisms may be due to three principal mechanisms: (1) reduction in neutrophil numbers (neutropenia), (2) a deficiency in opsonisation or (3) an inherited disorder affecting a specific neutrophil activity. The two general mechanisms which may cause neutropenia (as well as the reduction of other cellular components of blood) are decreased or ineffective production and increased destruction. The most common causes of production failure are bone marrow suppression by irradiation or cytotoxic drugs, idiosyncratic drug

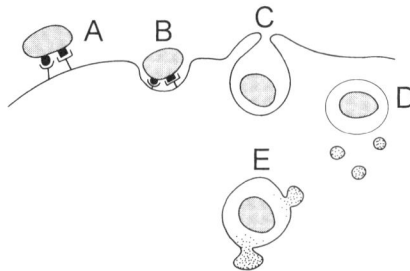

Figure 8 Phagocytosis. A: Bacterium opsonised with antibody and complement becomes attached to receptors on neutrophil cell membrane. B: Membrane invaginates. C: Phagosome is formed. D: Reactive oxygen species produced. E: Phagosome fuses with granules (lysosomes) to form phagolysosome. Bacterium is digested.

reactions (affecting only a very small number of patients taking those drugs) and various viral infections. In addition, vitamin deficiency (B_{12} and folate) and primary marrow failure may impede neutrophil production. Increased destruction of neutrophils is mostly caused by auto-antibody production, which may be secondary to drugs or occur in association with autoimmune diseases such as systemic lupus erythematosus (SLE) (page 201).

Opsonisation defects may result from deficiency of either antibody or complement. Complement deficiency may be inherited or acquired. Loss of complement components involved in the early part of the activation process (C2) is associated with autoimmune disease (e.g. SLE). Loss of the middle components (C3 or C5) results in an increased risk of pyogenic infection. Loss of later components of the complement cascade (C6, C7 or C8) results in a specific susceptibility to meningitis due to *Neisseria meningitidis*.

Failure to generate reactive oxygen species will impair neutrophil function and occurs as a result of several rare inherited enzyme defects. Loss of H_2O_2 production is caused by a deficiency of NADPH oxidase leading to chronic granulomatous disease. This affects macrophages as well as neutrophils. Affected infants are susceptible to recurrent infections, developing both multiple abscesses and granulomas.

MONOCYTES AND MACROPHAGES

Although monocytes are regarded as chronic inflammatory cells (see Chapters 13 and 14), they appear early in the course of acute inflammation and their extravasation into the tissues at the site of infection or injury is mediated by the same mechanism as that described for neutrophils. Outside the vascular compartment, the monocyte transforms into a larger phagocytic cell or macrophage. The macrophage has a much longer half-life than a neutrophil and is highly efficient at phagocytosis. Nitric oxide (generated within macrophages from the amino acid arginine) is a cytotoxic free radical which facilitates the killing of micro-organisms but also results in tissue damage (Lowenstein & Snyder, 1992).

EOSINOPHILS

In tissue sections eosinophils typically have a bilobed nucleus and large, brightly eosinophilic cytoplasmic granules. The granules contain a variety of enzymes which are released upon provocation. Eosinophils also secrete inflammatory mediators such as leukotrienes and platelet activating factor (see below). Eosinophils appear to have a variety of functions but are particularly effective as a defence against parasitic worms. They are also associated with hypersensitivity reactions, fungal infections and granulomatous inflammation.

BASOPHILS AND MAST CELLS

Basophils and mast cells develop from the same precursor cell, the former being intravascular and the latter located in either connective tissues or the mucosal lining of hollow organs. The basophilic granules contain histamine, heparin and additional inflammatory mediators. Mast cells are able to synthesise inflammatory mediators *de novo*, such as prostaglandins. The mast cell is implicated in type I (immediate) hypersensitivity (page 89).

PLASMA ENZYME SYSTEMS

Complement

This complex enzyme system is driven by a cascade mechanism through a 'classical' pathway (activated by immune complexes) and an 'alternative' pathway (activated by micro-organisms). The main reactive products are C3b, involved in opsonisation of micro-organisms, and C5a, which is a powerful inflammatory mediator that increases vascular permeability and serves as a neutrophil chemotaxin. Complement is a crucial component of the host's natural defences to infection.

Kinins

Kinins are derived from circulatory precursors called kallikreins and cause vasodilation and increased vascular permeability. Bradykinin stimulates pain receptors.

Coagulation factors

Coagulation factors are discussed in Chapter 17. The formation of fibrin serves to entrap micro-organisms and so facilitate phagocytosis.

OTHER INFLAMMATORY MEDIATORS

Histamine

Major sites of storage of histamine are mast cells and platelets. The principal effects of histamine in acute inflammation include vasodilation, increased vascular permeability and neutrophil chemotaxis.

Eicosanoids and platelet activating factor (PAF)

These do not exist as preformed chemicals but are synthesised by activated inflammatory cells from the fatty acid arachidonic acid. The latter is released from cell membrane phospholipids by the action of phospholipase A_2. There are two main families of eicosanoids: prostaglandins and leukotrienes. The prostaglandins have multiple biological effects, both stimulating and inhibiting inflammation. The ability of aspirin and other non-steroidal anti-inflammatory drugs to suppress inflammation is explained in part by their inhibition of the enzyme cyclo-oxygenase (which converts arachidonic acid to prostaglandin G_2). Leukotrienes are powerful inflammatory mediators serving as neutrophil chemotaxins and causing increased vascular permeability.

PAF, like the eicosanoids, is not stored in inflammatory cells but synthesised upon cell activation. As well as causing platelet aggregation, PAF increases vascular permeability, serves as a chemotaxin and helps to activate neutrophils and macrophages.

CYTOKINES

The interleukins (IL) are a large family of chemical mediators and messengers produced by white blood cells. IL-1 is produced by monocytes and macrophages. Amongst its many functions are neutrophil recruitment and activation. Interferons are notable for their ability to inhibit viral replication. Tumour necrosis factor-α (TNF-α) has numerous functions relating to both inflammatory and immune responses. It acts with IL-1 to induce the expression of neutrophil and endothelial adhesion molecules and activation of neutrophils.

In summary, pyogenic bacteria trigger a host response by: (1) penetrating the host's natural defences, (2) multiplying in a normally protected environmental niche, (3) producing a specific pattern of tissue injury, and (4) causing the release of inflammatory mediators which orchestrate the recruitment and activation of phagocytic neutrophils. The accompanying tissue changes are described in the following chapter.

REFERENCES

Lachmann, P.J. (1992) Complement. In *Oxford Textbook of Pathology*, volume 1, edited by J.O'D. McGee, P.G. Isaacson & N.A. Wright, pp. 259–266. Oxford: Oxford University Press.

Lowenstein, C.J. & Snyder, S. (1992) Nitric oxide, a novel biologic messenger. *Cell*, **70**, 705–707.

Savill, J.S., Wyllie, A.M., Henson, J.E., Walport, M.J., Henson, P.M. & Haslett, C. (1989) Macrophage phagocytosis of aging neutrophils in inflammation. Programmed cell death in the neutrophil leads to its recognition by macrophages. *J Clin Invest,* **83**, 865–875.

Further reading

Pace-Asciak, C. & Granstrom, E. (1983) Prostaglandins and related substances. *New Comprehensive Biochemistry*, volume 5. Amsterdam: Elsevier.

Willoughby, D.A. (1987) Inflammation–mediators and mechanisms. *British Medical Bulletin*, vol 43, no. 2. London: Churchill Livingstone.

TISSUE RESPONSES TO INFECTION AND INJURY

Your son, corporal Frank H. Irwin, was wounded near Fort Fisher, Virginia, March 25, 1865. The wound was in the left knee, pretty bad ... On the 4th of April the leg was amputated a little above the knee – the operation was performed by Dr. Bliss, one of the best surgeons in the army ... There was a good deal of bad matter gathered — the bullet was found in the knee. The last ten or twelve days of April I saw that his case was critical. He previously had some fever, with cold spells. He died 1st of May. The actual cause of death was pyaemia, the absorption of the matter in his system instead of its discharge

Walt Whitman, 1865 (*Specimen Days – Death of a Pennsylvania Soldier*)

Why are acutely inflamed tissues red and swollen?

INTRODUCTION

We usually take the body's defences against infection or injury for granted, not realising that potential pathogens are being repelled successfully on a continuous basis and before they have a chance to provoke a noticeable response. Some micro-organisms, particularly viruses, may initiate an immune response that is not accompanied by symptoms of any kind. This is termed a subclinical infection. It is also common, again mainly with certain types of virus, for infection to lie latent within the body, reawakening in response to a stimulus or to immune suppression. Viruses achieve this dormant state by integrating their own DNA with that of the host. Some bacteria, notably *Mycobacterium tuberculosis*, may also lie dormant for years. This chapter will be confined to a general overview of the major types of clinically apparent tissue response evoked by infective or injurious agents.

ACUTE INFLAMMATORY REACTION

The cellular and humoral mechanisms underlying the acute inflammatory reaction have been considered in Chapter 12 and provide the basis for the classical description by Celsus. Rubor (redness) and calor (heat) are due to vasodilation and increased blood flow (caused initially by histamine and then maintained by a variety of inflammatory mediators). Tumour, or swelling, is caused by the outpouring of plasma from leaky vessels (bathing the infected site with antibodies and complement). Dolor (pain) results from the stretching of swollen tissues as well as the inflammatory mediators of pain, specifically bradykinin and prostaglandins. The production of 'matter' or pus (suppuration) alluded to in the quotation above refers to the inflammatory exudate comprising dead and dying neutrophils. The discharge of pus (whether spontaneous or surgical) was understood to presage recovery. The inflammatory exudate varies according to the proportion of cells and plasma proteins. A serous exudate is straw coloured with abundant protein but few cells. A fibrinous exudate is associated with excessive deposition of fibrin. A purulent exudate is rich in pus. Exudation into a serous cavity (such as a pleural sac) is called an effusion.

The features of acute inflammation are reproduced faithfully in all the tissues of the body and are most dramatic when the underlying cause is infection with pyogenic (pus-generating) bacteria. Examples are staphylococcal skin infections, meningitis, appendicitis and pneumonia. The natural history of acute pyogenic inflammation is well illustrated by pneumonia caused by *Streptococcus pneumonia* (pneumococcus) in which a distinct ordering of tissue changes occurs with time (as shown by the autopsy examination of the lungs of subjects dying at various stages). The stages are: (1) congestion, (2) red hepatisation, (3) gray hepatisation, and (4) resolution.

Congestion

The lung is heavy, fluid laden and red. The tissue counterparts are engorgement of the intra-alveolar capillaries and venules and the outpouring of a protein rich inflammatory exudate into the alveoli. Bacteria are present, sometimes in large numbers.

Red hepatisation

The lung is red and heavy and solid and resembles liver (first noted by Morgagni). The solidity or consolidation is due to the exudation of red blood cells into alveoli and the intra-alveolar conversion of soluble fibrinogen into fibrin. The latter entraps bacteria and intra-alveolar neutrophils are actively phagocytic.

Grey hepatisation

There is continued outpouring by neutrophils into the alveoli whereas the red blood cells are lysed. Hence the lung appears grey and remains firm or consolidated. The conversion of fibrinogen to fibrin results in a relatively dry cut surface when the lung is sectioned. In the pre-antibiotic era this was the stage of crisis. Either the patient would die or there would be resolution by lysis (accompanied by profuse sweating and a sustained lowering of body temperature).

Resolution

The inflammatory exudate is converted to granular debris under the influence of enzymatic digestion. Debris and dead neutrophils are phagocytosed by macrophages. Some of the debris is absorbed and some is coughed up. Ultimately there may be complete restoration of normal lung architecture. In classical lobar pneumonia, the inflammatory exudate spreads like a wave (via alveolar pores of Kohn) throughout the affected lung lobe, producing diffuse consolidation. The overlying pleura is typically covered by a shaggy fibrinous exudate (pleurisy or pleuritis).

Complications of acute inflammation

The most desirable outcome of an acute inflammatory reaction is elimination of the cause followed by complete restoration of normal structure and function. However, this does not always come about. The main complications of acute inflammation are: (1) fibrosis, (2) abscess formation, (3) bacterial dissemination to distant sites, (4) progression to chronic inflammation, (5) secondary ischaemia leading to tissue necrosis and (6) formation of sinuses or fistulae.

Fibrosis

The term fibrosis means the laying down of collagen-rich connective tissue. Fibrosis occurs either in response to tissue destruction (see below) or when there is excessive deposition of fibrin. The process whereby fibrin (or thombus or dead tissue) is removed and replaced by connective tissue is called organisation. In the lung, fibrosis may occur within the alveoli, converting the normal air-filled, sponge-like parenchyma into useless and solid flesh-like tissue (carnification). In the pleural sac, the visceral and parietal leaves will become thickened and mutually adherent. Fibrous adhesions affecting the serosal membrane of the gut may lead to gut obstruction as a result of twisting or kinking of bowel loops.

Abscess formation

An abscess is a localised collection of pus. It arises on the basis of liquefactive tissue necrosis caused by the excessive release of hydrolytic and proteolytic enzymes and cytotoxic inflammatory mediators by neutrophils and macrophages. The wall of an abscess is lined by granulation tissue, a loose reactive layer of connective tissue comprising capillaries, fibroblasts laying down collagen and inflammatory cells. With time, the amount of collagen in the wall increases to give rise to a chronic abscess. Purulent effusions within particular spaces of the abdominal cavity are referred to as abscesses, particularly when they become walled off.

Bacterial dissemination

Bacteria may spread from the primary site of infection to give rise to metastatic infection. This is facilitated when an infected thrombus is carried from the site as an embolism (see Chapter 18) which then lodges in the miscrovasculature of the target tissue.

Progression to chronic inflammation

This occurs when the cause of the acute inflammatory reaction persists, or the process of healing cannot be brought to completion. Chronic inflammation is discussed below.

Ischaemic injury

The sluggish flow in the inflamed microvasculature and the release of inflammatory mediators leads to platelet aggregation, thrombosis and vascular occlusion (see Chapter 17). On top of this, the tissue oedema interferes with the arterial supply of the affected part and ischaemic necrosis may ensue. Superadded bacterial infection results in gangrene (the combination of necrosis and bacterial infection). In the appendix, for example, the result will be perforation leading to peritonitis.

Sinuses and fistulae

An inflammatory process may be connected to an epithelial surface by a track which discharges exudate that may be serous or purulent. A sinus is a blind-ending track, whereas a fistula connects two epithelial surfaces. Both are lined by granulation tissue. Failure to heal may be the result of infection, foreign material (such as hair in the case of a pilonidal sinus), the constant flow of luminal contents through an intestinal fistula or (more rarely) an underlying malignancy.

CHRONIC INFLAMMATION

As already stated, the term chronic refers to the duration of an inflammatory process persisting for months, years or even a lifetime. Chronic inflammation may be likened to a situation of stalemate between the forces of destruction and repair. Superimposed upon this state will be active or acute inflammation. Sometimes this is minimal or quiescent. The disease is then in remission. Periodically there may be bursts of active inflammation known as a state of relapse.

Certain types of infective agent cause chronic inflammation, for example *Mycobacterium tuberulosis* and *Treponema pallidum* (the cause of syphilis). Such organisms resist complete elimination by the immune system and provoke cell-mediated or delayed hypersensitivity (page 89). Other causes of chronic inflammation are non-degradable foreign material, long-term exposure to environmental irritants and autoimmune disease (Chapter 30).

The macrophage is a key cell in the mediation of chronic inflammation. In acute inflammation this cell plays a phagocytic role. Under the influence of T cell cytokines (e.g. interferons), the macrophage is transformed into an activated cell with enhanced phagocytic activity and the ability to synthesise its own cytokines (interleukin-1 (IL-1), tumor necrosis factor-α (TNF-α), fibroblast growth factor (FGF), transforming growth factor β (TGFβ), platelet derived growth factor (PDGF)), promoting fibrosis, angiogenesis and connective tissue remodelling. T lymphocytes are in turn activated by the production of IL-1, thereby completing a reciprocal state of activation. Although chronic inflammation is orchestrated by macrophages and T lymphocytes, other inflammatory cells, including plasma cells, eosinophils and neutrophils, are well represented.

Repair

Repair or healing may be an outcome of: (1) acute inflammation, (2) chronic inflammation, (3) necrosis (e.g. ischaemic) and (4) wounds and bone fractures. The principles underlying the repair process are similar in all four conditions. If the connective tissue framework of the tissue has not been destroyed and the tissue is not formed of permanent cells (incapable of division), regeneration is possible. This implies complete restoration of normal structure and function. This may occur in acute inflammatory conditions such as lobar pneumonia, in a skin wound and with respect to a bone fracture. When there has been more extensive tissue destruction, healing results in fibrosis or the permanent substitution of normal tissue by a fibrous scar.

Chronic peptic ulcer

A good example of healing by fibrosis is seen in a chronic peptic ulcer of the stomach or duodenum (Fig. 9). Ulceration implies loss of the surface epithelium, but the loss of normal tissue is far greater than this in a chronic peptic ulcer. The ulcer crater is covered with inflammatory exudate including dead neutrophils and below these a layer of fibrin. Beneath the fibrin is granulation tissue, and the remainder of the wall is made up of a fibrous scar. No normal tissue remains. The structure of a chronic ulcer is essentially the same as the wall of a chronic abscess. The epithelium may ultimately regenerate and cover the ulcer crater but the underlying scar tissue will persist.

Wound healing

In the case of a skin wound, the defect is filled by plasma which coagulates to form a scab. The epithelium regenerates beneath the scab. Below this is granulation tissue which may be visualised directly in a large cutaneous wound that has not scabbed over. It appears as a red, delicate and granular membrane. Granulation tissue provides nutritional support through its proliferated new thin-walled vessels, inflammatory cells to combat infection and phagocytose debris, fibroblasts to lay down collagen and macrophages to stimulate fibroblastic activity and coordinate the laying down and subsequent remodelling of scar tissue. In larger wounds that have not been sutured (healing by secondary as opposed to primary intention), contraction of the wound occurs through the activity of myofibroblasts. These hybrid cells synthesise collagen but are also able to link up and contract via their cytofilaments of smooth muscle actin. In this way the sides of the wound are brought together by natural mechanisms.

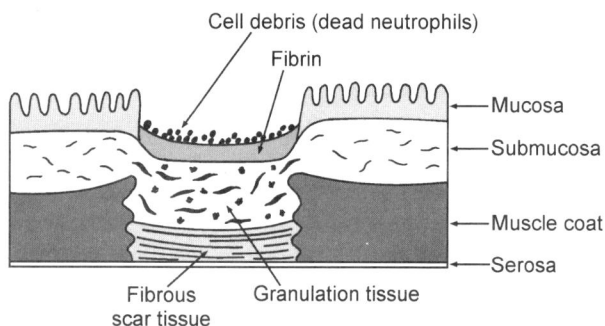

Figure 9 Structure of a chronic peptic ulcer of the stomach

Collagen

The extracellular matrix of granulation tissue and fibrous tissue comprises several types of extracellular protein. The most important of these in terms of its quantity and tensile strength is collagen. There are different types of collagen, some forming fibrils with a distinct architectural structure at the electron microscope level and others being amorphous. Type I collagen is fibrillary and is the most common type, being found in skin, bone, tendon and scar tissue produced in the course of healing. At the electron microscopic level, type I collagen consists of bundles of fibres with regular transverse bands. Basement membrane type IV collagen, by contrast, is amorphous.

Collagen is synthesised in the form of three alpha chains entwined in a helix. A key step in this process is the hydroxylation of the amino acid proline requiring the presence of vitamin C. Vitamin C deficiency will therefore delay wound healing. Other factors inhibiting wound healing include mechanical interference, infection, foreign material and steroid use. The procollagen is then crosslinked (outside the fibroblast) to form collagen fibrils. Tensile strength within a wound is a factor of both the amount and structural orientation of the collagen fibres. Remodelling is an active process involving both synthesis and controlled degradation of collagen. Degradation is achieved by a family of zinc-dependent enzymes called metalloproteinases, which are synthesised by fibroblasts, inflammatory cells and some epithelial cells. Metalloproteinase activity is controlled by a further family of enzymes called tissue inhibitors of metalloproteinase (TIMP). Expression of metalloproteinases is thought to be a key step in the early invasion of cancer, which involves the degradation of extracellular matrix proteins. A cancer may therefore be described as a wound that never heals.

Granulomatous inflammation

Granulomatous inflammation may be viewed as a variant of chronic inflammation in which activated macrophages group together to form aggregates, or granulomas (Fig. 10). At the same time the macrophages transform into non-motile epithelioid cells. The name epithelioid is derived from the fact that the cells have an abundant, but rather indistinct eosinophilic cytoplasm, and resemble epithelial cells. Granulomas may range from microscopic collections of epithelioid cells (microgranulomas) to larger lesions, visible macroscopically as pale nodules. In tuberculosis, the latter are described as tubercles (from which the term tuberculosis is

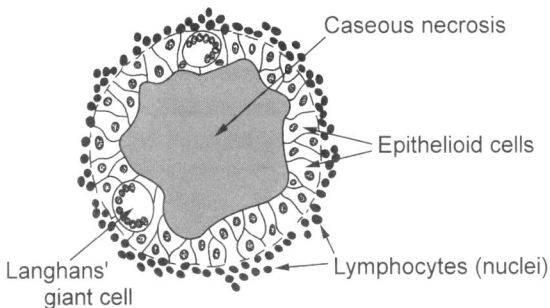

Figure 10 Tuberculous granuloma with central caseous necrosis

derived). A single large tumour-like tuberculous granuloma is called a tuberculoma.

Granulomas are typically surrounded by a rim of activated T lymphocytes, the lymphocytes and epithelioid cells being in a state of mutual activation through the release of cytokines. With increasing age, and through the synthesis of fibrogenic growth factors by the epithelioid cells, granulomas may develop a rim of connective tissue. The epithelioid cells often fuse to form giant cells of which two main types are recognised: foreign body giant cells, with haphazardly arranged nuclei, and Langhans' giant cells in which the nuclei are arranged in a peripheral wreath (Fig. 11). Langhans' giant cells, are a characteristic component of tuberculous granulomas.

A key hallmark of the tuberculous granuloma is the presence of caseous necrosis, so named because of its macroscopic likeness to soft, white cheese. Microscopically, the caseous necrosis occupies the centre of the granuloma and stains as amorphous pink material. Caseous necrosis is rare in granulomas associated with other conditions.

Causes of granulomatous inflammation other than tuberculosis include bacterial infections (such as syphilis, leprosy, brucellosis and cat-scratch disease), parasitic worms, fungal infections, inorganic material (silica and beryllium), sarcoidosis, Crohn's disease and non-degradable foreign material. This list of common causes is fairly limited (in fact, there is a longer list of more uncommon possibilities), and the diagnosis of a granuloma narrows down the possible causes of chronic inflammation considerably. Common to all these conditions are organisms or foreign materials that are poorly degradable. This is often coupled with enhanced T cell-mediated immunity (see Chapter 14).

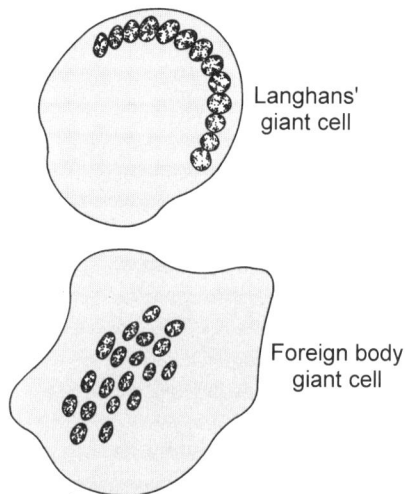

Figure 11 Giant cells: Langhans' and foreign body types

REFERENCES

Further reading

Majno, G. (1979) The story of the myofibroblasts. *Am J Surg Pathol,* **3**, 535–542.

Matrisian, L.M. (1992) The matrix-degrading metalloproteinases. *Bioassays,* **14**, 455–463.

Piezm K.A. & Reddi, A.H. (1984) *Extracellular Matrix Biochemistry.* New York: Elsevier.

Schilling, J.A. (1976) Wound healing. *Surg Clin North Am,* **56**, 859–874.

Thomas, R. & Lipsky, P.E. (1993) Monocytes and macrophages. In *Textbook of Rheumatology* (4th edn), volume 1, edited by W.N. Kelly et al., pp. 286–303. Philadelphia: Saunders.

— 14 —

INFLAMMATION AND
THE IMMUNE SYSTEM

*Ignorance of the function of the lymphocyte is one of
the most disgraceful gaps in our medical knowledge*

Arnold R. Rich (1936)

How do antibodies recognise antigens?

SPECIFIC IMMUNITY

As noted in Chapter 12, the body's system of defence against pathogenic micro-organisms
can be subdivided into two principal categories:

1. Natural immunity that does not require previous exposure to the pathogen. The inflammatory reaction is non-specific, meaning that it is broadly similar regardless of the underlying cause.
2. Specific or acquired immunity in which the immune system responds in a specific manner to the causative agent and retains a memory of the encounter.

The two forms of immunity are complementary and may be observed working together to
combat many infective processes. For example, phagocytosis by neutrophils occurs with far
greater efficiency when the target microbe has been dressed with antibodies (the concept of
opsonisation dates back to 1903 and the work of Sir Almroth Wright). Furthermore, cells of
the monocyte lineage may function either in a non-specific manner as phagocytic macrophages
or as antigen presenting cells in the context of specific immunity. Therefore some of the
components of acquired immunity have been described in Chapter 12. In this chapter, the
structure and function of the immune system will be considered in more detail.

The two types of immunity are essential for survival. Although acute inflammation may
lead to complications that can be life-threatening (such as fibrous adhesions causing intestinal obstruction), these excesses are more a reflection of the virulence of the infective agent.
By contrast, the enormous complexity of specific immunity, while essential for the survival of
the species, introduces many opportunities for malfunction which may be disastrous for the

individual. The malfunction may take three forms: absent function, defective function or excessive function. The causes of malfunction may be genetic or environmental in origin, or a combination of the two.

OLD AND NEW IMMUNOLOGY

Divisions into 'old' and 'new' immunology were hinted at in Chapter 10. Old immunology was utilitarian, but based on simplistic concepts. The focus was on vaccines, antitoxins and serum-based factors. Cellular mechanisms did not extend beyond phagocytosis. Nevertheless, the practical results were spectacular. New immunology turned to the underlying structure and function of the immune system as a whole. Based upon rigorous scientific research extending over the last forty years, new immunology has yielded much understanding but this has not yet been translated into therapeutic benefits to match those of the old immunology.

Before considering the subject of the quotation, the lymphocyte, the pioneering concepts by Burnet and Medawar must be introduced. Up until 1949 it was believed that the information required to produce an antibody was contained within the antigen. In other words the antigen served as the template. An original idea put forward by Burnet and Fenner in 1949 turned this view around completely. They realised that the old theory was deficient because it did not explain why organisms fail to produce antibodies to their own antigens. Clearly there had to be a highly intelligent mechanism to allow an animal to distinguish 'self' from 'non-self'. Billingham, Brent and Medawar (1953) showed that the tolerance towards 'self' is acquired before birth. When foreign mouse cells were introduced into a mouse before birth, the mouse would later accept a skin graft from the donor animal. These observations allowed Burnet to discard the old template theory of antibody production and replace it with his clonal model. He envisaged a system in which the large repertoire of potential antibody structures is genetically predetermined. When an antigen is recognised by the immune system as being 'non-self', an immune cell capable of matching the structure of the antigen with an appropriate antibody will divide repeatedly to form a clone of identical cells producing the same antibody (Burnet, 1960).

ANTIBODIES

How is it possible to achieve preformed antibody production, given the seemingly unlimited range of antigenic structures that might invade a host? To answer this question it is necessary to present a brief account of the structure and synthesis of antibodies. The basic structure of an antibody or immunoglobulin was shown (by the 1972 Nobel prize winners Porter and Edelman) to comprise a four peptide unit made of two identical heavy chains (of which there are five classes: (γ, α, β, μ, δ and ϵ) and two identical light chains (of which there are two classes: κ and λ). These chains are assembled in the form of a pair of heavy chains as shown in Fig 12. This complex molecule is not coded for by a single gene but by clusters of genes on three different chromosomes (2, 11 and 14). The variable end of the molecule combines with an antigen. The variability arises because of a process in which germline DNA is rearranged into a simpler DNA template that is actually employed for transcription. For example, germline DNA contains over 70 V_k genes of which only one is used to generate the variable domain of a particular kappa light chain. Since heavy chains also have a variable end, the permutations of antigen-recognising structures are enormous. Once primed in this way, a potential antibody-secreting B cell expresses its own unique or signature immunoglobulin molecule upon its cell surface (as IgM). The fact of gene rearrangement is exploited for diagnostic purposes in ingenious ways, for example to demonstrate clonality and lineage in the case of malignant lymphomas.

Antibody production (seroconversion) is initiated when a B lymphocyte encounters an antigen with a complementary structure. During the primary response to a new antigen of infective origin, the affected subject may develop an illness. Should the same antigen be introduced later, the secondary response may be so efficient (because of B cell memory) that the individual suffers no ill-effects, i.e. has full immunity.

There are five immunoglobulin classes as determined by the type of heavy chain: IgG, IgA, IgM, IgD and IgE). Of the three classes occurring as monomers (IgG, IgD and IgE), IgG is the most plentiful. IgA exists as a dimer and is the major immunoglobulin in external secretions. IgM is a pentamer and the key to the primary immune response. IgE is unique in binding to mast cells and basophils and triggering the release of secretory granules containing histamine and other inflammatory mediators.

T LYMPHOCYTES

The immune system is now perceived as having both memory and intelligence and the intelligence resides at the level of the gene. In other words the antigen is merely a provocation; the response to it is genetically predetermined. By 1945 it had been known for decades that serum derived antibodies could be transferred from one animal to another and so transmit passive immunity. In that year Chase demonstrated that immunity could be transferred by means of lymphocytes. In 1960 Nowell showed that the circulating small round lymphocyte was not an endstage cell, but could be stimulated to transform into a blast cell capable of clonal expansion.

The separation of lymphocytes into T cells and B cells began through investigations of the thymus gland. Up until the 1960s the thymus gland was usually classed as an endocrine gland, yet its removal in both animals and humans (due to thymic cancer, for example) has no appreciable effect. The thymus is large in newborn humans and other newborn mammals,

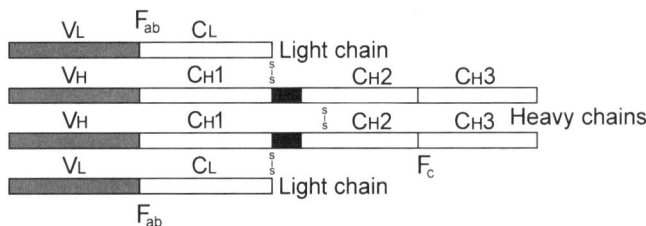

Figure 12 Antibody formed of two light chains and two heavy chains. These are linked by disulphide bonds. The variable domain of the chains binds to antigen. The effector end (F_c fragment) binds to leukocyte receptors or activates the complement cascade by the 'classical' pathway (when the antibody is complexed with an antigen).

reaches its maximum size at around puberty (though by then has become relatively small compared with other organs), and then undergoes progressive atrophy.

In 1961 Jacques Miller in London and Robert Good at the University of Minnesota showed that removal of the thymus in newborn mice and rabbits produced very definite results. The animals failed to generate the usual population of lymphocytes, failed to reject skin grafts and most died before the age of three months with wasting and viral infections. Nevertheless these animals were still able to produce antibodies. Miller went on to show that the thymus gland was indeed a type of endocrine gland because it was composed of hormone producing epithelial cells. He proved this by transplanting thymic tissue contained within a sealed millipore chamber into the peritoneal cavity of thymectomised mice. Cells could not get in or out, but hormones (a polypeptide hormone identified subsequently and called thymosin) could traverse the millipore filter and restore lymphocyte function. Even on its own, thymosin was shown to partially restore cell mediated immunity (Roitt, 1994).

B LYMPHOCYTES

While still a graduate student at Ohio State University, Bruce Glick removed a lymphoid organ called the bursa of Fabricius (found only in birds) from young chicks shortly after hatching (Glick et al., 1956). This resulted in a profound impairment of antibody mediated immunity and a deficiency of plasma cells responsible for antibody synthesis. Removal of the thymus (possessed by birds as well as mammals), on the other hand, resulted in the same type of disordered cell-mediated immunity that Miller had described in thymectomised mice (Warner & Szenberg, 1964). Additional research involving selective knockout of the two systems led to the conclusion that immunodeficiency could result from loss of the stem cells from which all immune and haematological cells are derived, or from loss of selected and more differentiated arms of this system: thymus-dependent T lymphocytes and bursa-dependent B lymphocytes.

B AND T LYMPHOCYTES AND NATURAL KILLER (NK) CELLS

It became apparent that B lymphocyte function was not entirely normal in thymectomised animals. Cooperation between the B and T lymphocyte systems was required for a fully operational B cell immune system. A description of the early research into this cooperation between T and B cells that was undertaken in England, USA and Australia is beyond the reach of this short introduction, but it culminated in the recognition of the bone marrow as the source of B lymphocytes in mammals (conveniently so, given the preexisting B designation for bursa of Fabricius). Moreover, it was evident that T lymphocytes regulated the processes governing the differentiation of B lymphocytes into antibody-secreting plasma cells. Some T lymphocytes (expressing the cell membrane marker CD4 amongst others) helped this process (helper cells) whereas others (expressing CD8) suppressed it (suppressor cells) (Fig. 13). CD8 cells were also shown to be cytotoxic and capable of killing target cells that expressed appropriate antigens (such as when infected by a virus). Lymphocyte interaction was achieved by the synthesis of lymphokines, a large family of polypeptides functioning as intercellular chemical messengers but over short distances (unlike the traditional hormone). Natural killer (NK) cells were a third class of null cells (neither B nor T) with cytotoxic activity.

MAJOR HISTOCOMPATIBILITY COMPLEX (MHC) AND HUMAN LEUKOCYTE ANTIGENS (HLA)

The major histocompatibility complex (MHC) and human leukocyte antigens (HLA) were discovered when it became apparent that the sera of multiparous women or of patients who had received multiple blood transfusions contained antibodies directed to cell surface antigens expressed by foreign white blood cells. In humans, the MHC genes are located on chromosome 6p (p stands for petit or short arm, q for long arm) and code for two major classes of molecule: HLA classes I and II. Class I MHC antigens are coded for by genes in three regions (A, B and C) of the MHC, giving rise to a heavy chain that is highly polymorphic. The antigen comprises a second, non-polymorphic chain, β_2-microglobulin. Class I antigens are expressed by all nucleated cells.

An important role of these antigens is to signal changes in 'self' to the immune system to allow, for example, tumour cells or cells infected by viruses to be eliminated (Doherty & Zinkernagel, 1975). Class II MHC antigens are coded for by three loci in the D region of the MHC complex (DP, DQ and DR). These have a more restricted expression, mainly on the cell membranes of B lymphocytes and cells of the monocyte and macrophage lineage (mononuclear phagocytes).

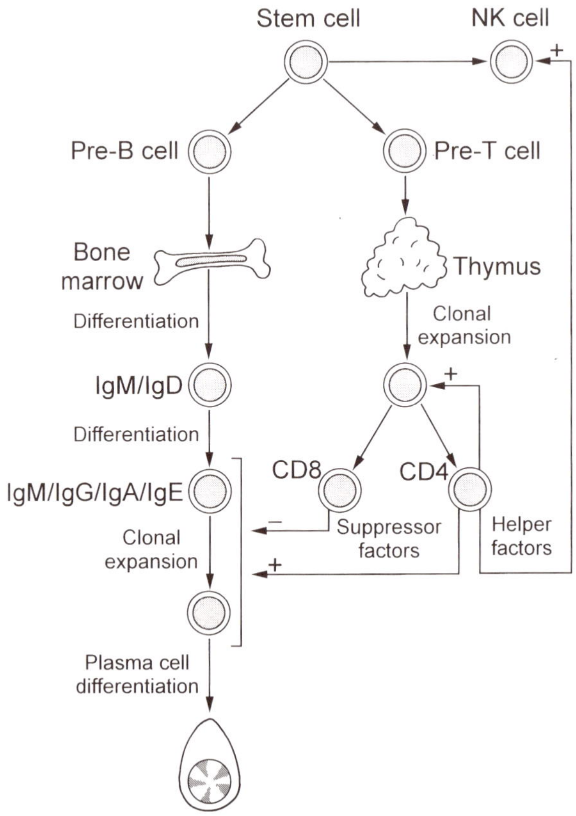

Figure 13 T and B lymphocyte arms of the specific immune system

MONOCYTES AND MACROPHAGES

The term mononuclear phagocyte encompasses a family of closely related cells that are given different names in different anatomical locations: monocytes in the blood, macrophages in the alveolar spaces of the lungs, histiocytes in interstitial tissues or in the sinuses of lymph nodes or spleen, Kupffer cells in the sinuses of the liver, osteoclasts in bone, dendritic cells in the T and B cell zones of lymphoid tissue (Fig. 14), Langerhans' cells in the skin and microglia in the brain. The system encompassing the sinuses of lymph nodes, spleen and liver was formerly known as the reticuloendothelial system. This unfortunate term has been replaced by the term mononuclear phagocytic system as it fails to describe the central cell lineage, its widespread distribution, or its many functions. Apart from ingesting antigenic material by the mechanism of phagocytosis, macrophages process and present the antigens on their cell membranes in conjunction with class II MHC antigens. The antigens may then elicit either a T or B cell response. Mononuclear phagocytes also secrete numerous chemical messengers (monokines) including interleukin-1 (IL-1) which has multiple functions (it promotes T cell function, catabolic metabolism and fever).

HYPERSENSITIVITY REACTIONS

An excessive response by the immune system to an antigenic stimulus that is damaging to the host is described as hypersensitivity. The antigen may be exogenous or derived from within the organism itself. The latter is described as autoimmunity and is discussed in Chapter 30. The Gell and Coombs classification of hypersensitivity reactions (Table 3) stems from the days of old immunology. Types I, III and IV hypersensitivity were described initially in 1902, 1905 and 1891 respectively (Bordley & Harvey, 1976). Only type IV hypersensitivity recognises the participation of the T lymphocyte. A single disease process may implicate two or more types of hypersensitivity. For example, types I, III and IV hypersensitivity are implicated in pulmonary aspergillosis (fungal infection) and types II and IV participate in antibody-dependent cellular cytotoxicity (ADCC). Type III hypersensitivity is responsible for most types of glomerulonephritis, yet this group of kidney disorders shows considerable

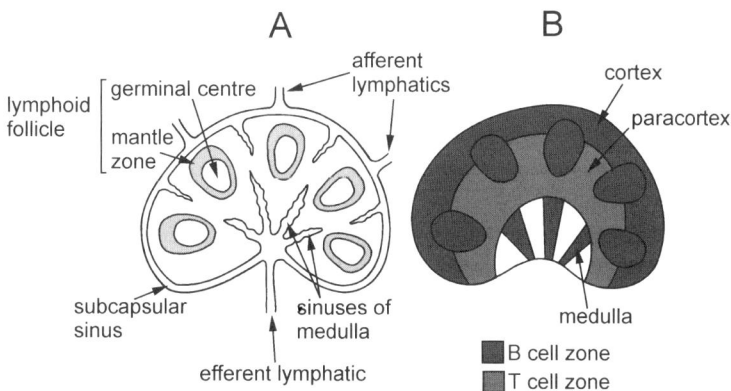

Figure 14 Lymph node: anatomical structure (A) and functional correlates (B)

variability in terms of morphology, natural history and prognosis. This is explained at least in part by the size and number of immune complexes bombarding the glomerulus. The classification of hypersensitivity given in Table 3 is therefore an oversimplification but still retains its popularity.

STRUCTURE OF THE LYMPHOID SYSTEM

Whilst the thymus and bone marrow may be perceived as the central elements of the immune system, most of the lymphocytes of the body are either circulating in the bloodstream or organised within specific anatomical structures: lymph nodes, spleen and mucosa associated lymphoid tissue (MALT) (e.g. tonsils and Peyer's patches in the terminal ileum). Because anatomy, haematology and immunology are traditionally taught as separate disciplines, students rarely perceive the connection between structure and function, and this impedes progression to an understanding of pathology. The B and T cell arms of the immune system converge upon the lymphoid tissue distributed in the anatomical locations noted above. Anatomical and functional correlates are shown for a lymph node in Figure 14 (page 89). It is within the tissues of the peripheral immune system that cells of the mononuclear phagocyte lineage present antigen to T and B cells, T cells instruct B cells, B cells transform into blasts (within the germinal centres of the lymphoid follicles) and B and T cells undergo clonal expansion.

Table 3 Classification of hypersensitivity reactions

Type	Mechanism	Examples
Type I (anaphylactic or immediate hypersensitivity)	Mast cells coated with IgE degranulate to release histamine	Hay fever, asthma, anaphylaxis
Type II (mediated by cytotoxic antibodies)	Cytotoxic antibodies (IgG or IgM) against self antigens. Complement is activated	Haemolytic anemia, Goodpastures syndrome, primary thyrotoxicosis
Type III (immune complex mediated)	Antibodies (IgG, IgM or IgA) formed against either extrinsic or intrinsic antigens result in circulating immune complexes. Neutrophils and complement contribute to tissue damage	Autoimmune diseases, glomerulonephritis, vasculitis
Type IV (cell mediated or delayed hypersensitivity)	Cooperation between T lymphocytes and macrophages mediated by interleukins and other cytokines	Tuberculosis, sarcoidosis, and other granulomatous disorders, many autoimmune diseases

IMMUNODEFICIENCY

Congenital forms

The congenital forms of immunodeficiency may implicate B cell function when there are repeated attacks of severe pyogenic infections (e.g. the X-linked Bruton type), T cell function (e.g. DiGeorge syndrome in which infants are born without a thymus and develop infections with viruses, fungi, protozoa and bacteria) and combined types (X-linked and recessive forms). The T and B cell zones of lymph nodes (Fig. 14) will be poorly represented in accord with the type of deficiency. Milder or more selective types of congenital immunodeficiency include common variable immunodeficiency (usually presenting in early adulthood), selective IgA deficiency and the X-linked Wiskott-Aldrich syndrome (presenting in the first few months of life and characterised by recurrent infections, eczema and thrombocytopenia in children).

ACQUIRED IMMUNODEFICIENCY SYNDROME (AIDS)

The acquired immunodeficiency syndrome (AIDS) is caused by infection of CD4 helper T cells by the human immunodeficiency virus (HIV). There is gradual depletion of this population and a resultant susceptibility to a variety of opportunistic infections (i.e. by organisms that are not normally pathogenic). There are four phases to the disease: (1) acute infection associated with seroconversion for the HIV antibody, (2) asymptomatic infection, (3) persistent generalised lymphadenopathy (lymph node enlargement), and finally (4) progression to AIDS. Common infections in AIDS include *Pneumocystis carinii*, Cytomegalovirus, *Candida* and other fungi, Herpes simplex, *Mycobacterium avium* complex and *Mycobacterium tuberculosis*. Additional manifestations are tumours (Kaposi's sarcoma and B cell lymphoma) and various disorders of the central and peripheral nervous systems.

Other forms of acquired immunodeficiency

Immunodeficiency may be acquired as a complication of administration of immunosuppressive drugs used to treat cancer or prevent graft rejection and a large variety of other conditions including infections, autoimmune disease, nephrotic syndrome, lymphoma and myeloma.

ANATOMICAL PATHOLOGY AND THE IMMUNE SYSTEM

The lymph nodes and extranodal mucosa associated lymphoid tissue (MALT) are important sites of pathology, particularly inflammation and neoplasia. Acute suppurative lymphadenitis affecting lymph nodes draining a site of bacterial infection is less common and less severe today than it was in the past because of the use of antibiotics. Such nodes enlarge rapidly, are tender and are associated with redness of the overlying skin. The term lymphadenopathy is truly warranted, but the same term is now often applied to nodes that are merely enlarged. A quinsy (again rare in the antibiotic era) is the same process involving the tonsils. Simple reactive hyperplasia of lymph nodes may implicate the B cell zones (hyperplasia of germinal centres and medullary cords), T cell zones (paracortex) and the mononuclear phagocytes (sinus histiocytosis). More specific inflammatory patterns are seen in tuberculosis, cat-scratch disease, toxoplasmosis, glandular fever and AIDS.

Tumours may include secondary deposits of carcinoma or melanoma, or primary neoplasms such as Hodgkin's disease or non-Hodgkin's lymphoma. Lymphomas of MALT (MALTomas) are biologically different to nodal lymphomas and are being diagnosed with increasing frequency. Diagnosis of these conditions requires knowledge of the limits of normal lymph node architecture and cytology. Diagnosis of non-Hodgkin's lymphoma has been aided by developments in new immunology. These include monoclonal antibodies to T and B cell markers and the molecular demonstration of gene rearrangement to prove both clonality (indicative of neoplasia) and cell lineage. Whilst diagnosis of lymphoma is precise, reflects the biological complexity of the immune system and carries prognostic significance, treatment options are still relatively limited.

AMYLOIDOSIS

Reference to amyloidosis is made in this chapter because of the frequent though by no means invariable association of this condition with disorders of the immune system. The term amyloid is applied to a heterogeneous group of proteins sharing the following features: (1) pink amorphous staining with H&E, (2) affinity for specific dyes such as Congo red and thioflavin T, and (3) apple-green birefringence when Congo red-stained amyloid is viewed microscopically under polarised light. Deposition of amyloid may either occur on a systemic basis, affecting organs such as the kidney, heart, liver, spleen, gastrointestinal tract and tongue, or be restricted to a single organ such as the brain or heart.

Amyloid is generally deposited in the connective tissues of organs in a diffuse manner. Severe amyloidosis results in enlargement of the affected organ, which appears pale when sectioned and is firm. The infiltrative process entraps the parenchymal cells, impedes their nutrition and ultimately leads to organ failure. The cut surface of an affected organ (viewed at autopsy, for example) stains with iodine (like starch). The word amyloid means starch-like, but the iodine is in fact staining a connective tissue molecule called glycosaminoglycan. Additionally, amyloid is made up of a fibrillary protein whose tertiary structure (β-pleated sheet) determines the staining characteristics described above. The actual nature of the amyloid polypeptide will be determined by the underlying cause. Regardless of the underlying cause, amyloid also includes a third constituent called amyloid P (AP).

Primary amyloidosis (the term primary implying merely that amyoidosis may be the first manifestation of the disease) occurs in a condition called multiple myeloma, which is a neoplasm of plasma cells associated with multiple foci of bone marrow involvement. The neoplastic plasma cells secrete immunoglobulin (IgG, IgA, IgD, IgE or IgM) or merely the kappa or lambda light chains of the immunoglobulin molecule. The amyloid protein is made of light chains (kappa or lambda) and is classified as AL. Chronic inflammation (e.g. rheumatoid arthritis and recurrent infection) causes secondary amyloidosis which is associated with an amyloid protein called AA. Secondary amyloidosis is now very uncommon because of the use of antibiotics to control infection, and immunosuppressive agents to treat autoimmune disorders. The terms 'primary' and 'secondary' are historical and no longer useful. Modern classifications are based on the precursor protein giving rise to amyloid. AA is also deposited in a primary familial form of amyloidosis called familial Mediterranean fever. Amyloidosis affecting synovial tissues and the gut complicates dialysis for chronic renal failure. The amyloid protein is classified as $A\beta_2m$ and is derived from β_2-microglobulin.

Single organ amyloidosis may accompany specific disorders such as Alzheimer's disease and Creutzfeld-Jakob disease of the brain, diabetes mellitus in which islet deposition is derived from amylin, and medullary carcinoma of the thyroid gland in which amyloid is generated from the polypeptide hormone calcitonin. Senile cardiac amyloid is derived from a serum protein called transthyretin (prealbumin) which transports thyroxine and retinol. This form of amyloidosis is usually asymptomatic. Senile amyloid deposition may also occur in the lungs and spleen.

Amyloidosis is not a single disease entity but a manifestation of a variety of disorders associated with protein deposition in interstitial tissues.

REFERENCES

Billingham, R.E., Brent, L. & Medawar, P.B. (1953) 'Actively acquired tolerance' of foreign cells. *Nature,* **172**, 603.

Bordley, J. III. & Harvey, A.M. (1976) *Two Centuries of American Medicine 1776–1976.* Philadelphia: Saunders.

Burnet, F.M. (1960) Theories of immunity. *Perspect Biol Med,* **3**, 447.

Doherty, P.C. & Zinkernagel, R.M. (1975) A biological role for the major histocompatibility antigens. *Lancet,* **i**, 1406.

Glick, B., Chang, J.S. & Jaap, R.C. (1956) The bursa of Fabricius and antibody production. *Poult Sci,* **35**, 224.

Roitt, I. (1994) *Essential Immunology* (8th edn), pp. 215–240. Oxford: Blackwell.

Warner, N.L. & Szenburg, A. (1964) Immunologic studies on normally bursectomized and surgically thymectomized chickens: Dissociation of immunologic responsiveness. In *The Thymus in Immununobiology,* edited by R.A. Good & A.E. Gabrielson, pp. 395–411. New York: Hoeber-Harper.

Further reading

Kisilevsky, R. (1994) Amyloidosis. *Pathology* (2nd edn), edited by E. Rubin & J.L. Farber, pp. 1163–1174. Philadelphia: JB Lippincott Co.

15

THE DIAGNOSIS OF INFLAMMATION: A PATHOLOGIST'S PERSPECTIVE

Truth cannot be concealed in the end

Leonardo da Vinci

What are the causes of inflammation?

INTRODUCTION

The distinction between cancer and non-cancer dominates the diagnostic work of the anatomical pathologist. The distinction may not be straightforward. Regeneration, inflammation and necrosis are features of cancer as well as innocent inflammatory processes. Conversely the altered appearances of reactive epithelial and connective tissue cells in inflammatory conditions can mimic those of cancer cells. As we have seen, inflammatory cells of the monocyte–macrophage lineage can group together into masses called granulomas (or tubercles in the case of tuberculosis). These were interpreted as tumours in the past and may still cause diagnostic difficulty. It should be recalled that the macrophages in granulomas are termed epithelioid cells because of their abundant eosinophilic cytoplasm. This explains the potential for confusion with epithelial malignancy. Stains used for studying bone marrow are excellent for distinguishing haematological cell types, but granulomas may be mistaken for epithelial malignancy in such preparations.

Once the distinction between a neoplastic and an inflammatory process has been made there is a tendency, if the condition is deemed to be inflammatory and apparently non-specific, for pathologists to draw a sigh of relief and take the matter no further. However, as appreciated by the Scottish anatomist and surgeon John Hunter (1728–93), inflammation is not a disease but a reaction. Whilst the tissues of the body have a limited repertoire of reactions to a vast range of noxious stimuli, it is helpful if the pathologist can find a specific cause for a 'non-specific' inflammatory response. In cases where the cause of an inflammatory disorder is unknown (this would apply to a large range of skin diseases) the 'pattern' of the inflammation will have diagnostic importance. The pattern is determined by the anatomical distribution of the inflammatory infiltrate, its severity, the cell types represented and the presence of additional features such as apoptosis, necrosis, blisters (in the case of skin) and disturbances of growth and differentiation of associated epithelial surfaces.

IDENTIFYING INFECTIVE AGENTS

The inflammation caused by micro-organisms may be out of all proportion to their number and size. Although bacteria may sometimes be visible in routine H&E sections, particularly when found in sizeable colonies, they are usually impossible to detect without the use of special stains, such as Gram for most bacteria and Ziehl-Neelsen for Mycobacteria species responsible for tuberculosis and related infections. Monoclonal antibodies to some bacteria, such as *Helicobacter pylori*, are also available for immunohistochemical or immunofluorescence staining. Even with the benefit of special stains, the pathologist must be prepared to search carefully for scanty micro-organisms. A single red-staining acid fast bacillus will confirm the presence of *Mycobacterium tuberculosis* but may require several minutes of observation using a high-power objective lens. Fungi may be equally scanty but will be visualised more easily when stained with periodic acid Schiff or silver techniques. Mycobacteria and fungi may be associated with a granulomatous reaction, and infiltrating eosinophils are often found in fungal infections.

Tissue may be sent to the laboratory in a fresh state deliberately to allow both microbiological isolation and characterisation (by microscopy, culture and sensitivity (MCS) to antibiotics) as well as histological examination. Microbiological techniques are more specific and sensitive than histological methods and fresh tissue should always be submitted to the laboratory when infection is included in the differential diagnosis. Molecular technology is increasingly being used to diagnose and classify micro-organisms, and serological testing

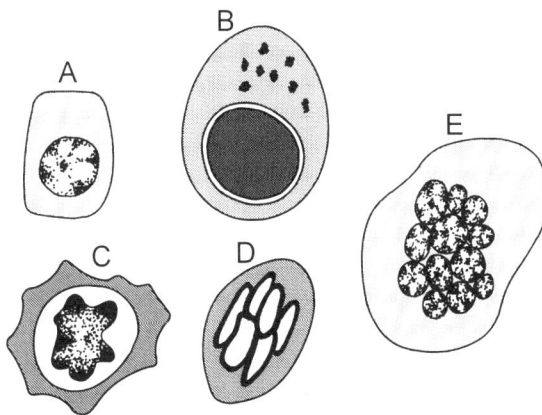

Figure 15 Direct viral cytopathic effects. A: Normal cell. B: Cytomegalovirus with large nuclear inclusion and cytoplasmic inclusions. C: Human papillomavirus. There is nuclear irregularity and cytoplasmic vacuolation (koilocytosis). D: Herpes virus with multinucleation. The nuclei contain homogeneous, 'ground-glass' inclusions (Cowdry B) and chromatin is compressed beneath the nuclear membrane. This virus also produces eosinophilic (Cowdry A) nuclear inclusions (not shown). E: Measles virus with multinucleation (Warthin-Finkeldey cell).

for specific antibodies also provides important diagnostic information.

Viruses are too small to be seen by the light microscope, but may produce pathological changes in cells (cytopathic effects) that are quite characteristic (Fig. 15). The changes include nuclear enlargement, irregularity and increased or reduced staining, cytoplasmic vacuolation, multinucleation and the presence of specific inclusions in the nucleus or cytoplasm. At the electron microscope level the latter will be seen as viral colonies and a specific diagnosis may be reached.

Parasites such as protozoa and worms may be readily seen with routine H&E sections. The eggs of worms are associated with the presence of tissue eosinophils and granulomatous inflammation.

DISORDERS OF IMMUNITY

The term 'hypersensitivity' implies a reaction by the immune defences that is excessive and results in inflammation that is detrimental to the host (see chapter 14). The stimulus may be a micro-organism, the antigenic products of micro-organisms, particular organic or inorganic matter or drugs. Hay fever and asthma are well-known types of hypersensitivity (type I) in which the mast cell triggers inflammation by releasing its granules containing histamine and heparin. In sensitised individuals, mast cells are coated with a type of antibody known as IgE. When the appropriate antigen is introduced, the IgE antibodies are activated and the mast cells degranulate. Mast cells are visualised by metachromatic dyes such as toluidine blue, which react with heparin sulphate. Eosinophils are attracted by the inflammatory mediators released by the mast cells.

Formation of immune complexes within the blood stream is another common type of hypersensitivity (type III). The complexes comprise antigen and antibody. When deposited within the walls of vessels (see chapter 19) complement is activated and this results in an acute inflammatory reaction in the vessel wall itself together with fibrin deposition (fibrinoid 'necrosis'). Destruction of the vessel wall results in the formation of haemorrhagic spots (described clinically as purpura when occurring in skin or mucous membranes). Vasculitis may be easily overlooked by the pathologist when the changes are mild and/or limited to a single small vessel.

Granulomatous inflammation may be viewed as a form of hypersensitivity as its extent is often disproportionate and destructive. Recognition of granulomatous inflammation (and its distinction from cancer) is important as it narrows down the list of possible aetiologies considerably. Granulomas may be overlooked when they are small, comprising no more than three or four epithelioid cells. Such microgranulomas are commonly seen in the liver and in Crohn's disease. Granulomas may also be loose and poorly formed, particularly in Crohn's disease. The most common causes of granulomas are listed on page 82. Foreign material is a common cause of granulomatous inflammation and may in some cases be detected by birefringence on polarised microscopy (the insertion of two polarising filters within the microscope's light beam).

REACHING A DIAGNOSIS

Inflammation may also be secondary to trauma (including self-inflicted trauma), heat, cold, chemical irritants, irradiation, ischemic necrosis and cancer. The likelihood of one cause over another will be influenced by the organ or system affected. Given the non-specific nature of many inflammatory reactions, the anatomical pathologist will need background information about the patient in order to assemble a reasonable set of working hypotheses. Age, gender, race, history of travel or of trauma, clinical signs, medical history and drug history may all be highly relevant, as will the findings of other special investigations, both laboratory-based and radiological. The diagnosis of 'non-specific inflammation' should become rarer and in-creasingly unacceptable with time.

REFERENCES

Further reading

Connor, D.H., Chandler, F.W., Schwartz, D.A., Manz, H.J. & Lack, E.E. (1997) *Pathology of Infectious Diseases*, volumes 1 and 2. Stamford, Connecticut: Appleton & Lange.

16

DISORDERS OF GROWTH
AND DIFFERENTIATION

The most incomprehensible thing about the universe is that it is comprehensible

Albert Einstein

What is differentiation?

LIFE CYCLE OF THE CELL

Growth and differentiation are normal properties of cells and tissues that are modified, disturbed or subverted in all disease states. Cancer could be described as the most extreme example of a disorder of growth and differentiation. Alternatively this disease may be viewed primarily as a disorder of the altered gene (see Chapter 23) that triggers multiple modifications of both cell structure and behaviour. In order to understand the changes in growth and differentiation that occur not only in cancer but in all diseases, it is necessary to appreciate normal structural and functional relationships as well as the underlying control mechanisms operating at the levels of molecules, cells and tissues. This is, of course, a topic of considerable magnitude. In this chapter it will only be possible to provide a glimpse of what is one of the most exciting and rapidly developing fields of biomedical research.

Cell function is divided into three broad categories: (1) proliferation, (2) death, and (3) differentiation. Cell proliferation focuses on the cell cycle (mitogenesis) and the mechanisms that initiate and control this process. Cell death implies the programmed demise of individual cells known as apoptosis. The balance of cell generation and cell death will determine whether an organ grows, shrinks or remains the same size. Differentiation is concerned with the control of gene induction which will provide a cell with its repertoire of housekeeping requirements as well as its specialised functions. Although proliferation, death and differentiation must be studied in isolation, because each is extraordinarily complex, they are integrated not only at the level of the cell but also at the level of tissues. The global orchestration of proliferation, death and differentiation is encountered in its most dynamic and extraordinary form during embryological development. However the *Hox* genes, which are restricted to the animal kingdom and occur in clustered arrays for sequential activation of target genes during embryological development, also function in the stem cells of adult tissues. This is one of many examples of a single gene having multiple functions. The following account of the proliferation, death and differentiation of cells will include issues that are of particular interest to the anatomical pathologist because of their practical importance in tissue diagnosis.

PROLIFERATION

Only certain adult tissues, described as labile, show continuous cell proliferation. These include the skin, the epithelial lining of the gut and respiratory tract, the endometrium, bone marrow, germinal centres of secondary lymphoid follicles in lymph nodes and seminiferous tubules of the testis. These tissues are at particular risk of both cancer and radiation damage. Other adult tissues do not normally divide but will do so when stimulated by either physiological or pathological factors. Examples of such stable tissues are liver, kidney, endocrine glands and smooth muscle. Cells that show essentially no capacity to divide in adult life (permanent cell populations) include neurons, cardiac muscle and skeletal muscle fibres. Cancers very rarely arise in permanent tissues, particularly in adults.

In labile tissues, a colony or patch (clone) is maintained by a single stem cell. A stem cell is self-generating. When it divides, one descendant takes the place of the stem cell and the other gives rise to daughter cells. The immediate descendants of a stem cell may be able to differentiate into two or more different lineages, but after a few divisions such multipotentiality is lost. Committed cells showing early maturation towards their end (terminal) state retain the capacity to divide, but eventually proliferation ceases and cytoplasmic maturation takes over. Finally the cell dies (by apoptosis) and is either phagocytosed or shed (Fig. 16).

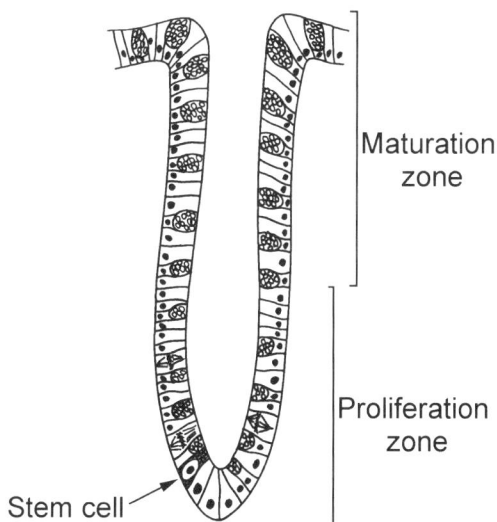

Figure 16 Normal colonic crypt. This is a clonal unit maintained by a single stem cell. The crypt is lined by goblet cells, columnar cells and scattered endocrine cells (not shown). Cells are generated in the proliferative compartment and migrate upwards to complete their cycle of maturation within a few days.

Cell division is a remarkable process. It is just as remarkable as returning to a book that one has placed upon a bookshelf the day before and finding a perfect replica sitting next to the original. Cell division involves a resting phase (G_1), a phase of synthesising DNA (S), a preparatory phase for mitosis (G_2) and finally mitosis (M) (Fig. 17). The commencement of each active step in the cell cycle (DNA synthesis and mitosis) is dependent upon the satisfactory completion of the previous step. 'Checkpoints' are regulatory pathways that oversee the dependence of one process on the previous one (Kaufmann & Paules, 1996). If a process is not completed satisfactorily, the checkpoint mechanism recognises this fact and blocks further progression until the fault is rectified. If the fault is very serious, the checkpoint mechanism may signal programmed cell death or apoptosis (page 102). Checkpoint dysfunction can result either in genetic mutation (for example through inactivation of the G_1 checkpoint genes *Rb* or *p53*), or in alterations in chromosomal number or structure through mutation of mitotic checkpoint genes (Cahill et al., 1998). Checkpoint dysfunction leads to a state of genetic instability (hypermutability) which underlies the pathogenesis of many types of cancer (see Chapter 23).

Cell division must be coordinated with the needs of tissue and indeed the entire organism. This is achieved by means of hormones and growth factors, hormone and growth factor receptors arranged upon the cell membrane, signal transduction pathways (transferring messages from cell membrane to nucleus) and nuclear proteins (to prepare the cell for division). The function of signal transduction pathways is to bring about amplification and integration of the various messages received by the array of receptors upon the cell surface and so relay an unambiguous message to the nucleus. These cascade systems operate through the enzymatic conversion of an inactive precursor to an active enzyme. This is achieved by a surprisingly limited number of mechanisms (Fig. 18). Some of the genes coding for growth factors, receptors, cell signalling molecules or nuclear proteins that drive mitogenesis are called proto-oncogenes. This is because mutated versions (oncogenes; see Chapter 23) have been shown to drive cell proliferation in neoplasms (Table 4).

Cell division is utilised by the anatomical pathologist for diagnostic purposes, particularly in relation to neoplasia. The presence of mitoses and the presence of abnormal mitoses are used to diagnose cancer. Mitotic counts are also employed to grade certain types of cancer (Chapter 22). Because the mitotic phase of the cell cycle is relatively short, estimates of proliferation have to be based upon a small number of observations. Nuclear proteins (PCNA and Ki-67) expressed during the cell cycle can be stained with specific monoclonal

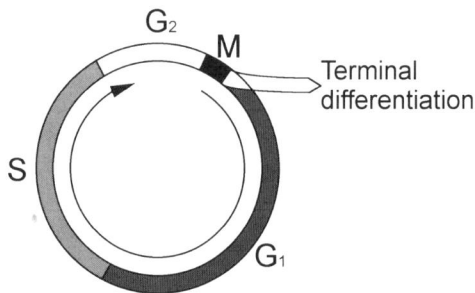

Figure 17 The cell cycle. G_1: gap 1; G_2: gap 2; M: mitotic phase; S: DNA synthetic phase. The entire cycle is completed in a matter of hours.

Table 4 Proto-oncogenes involved in carcinogenesis

Proto-oncogene	Function	Mechanism of activation	Sites or types of cancer
c-sis	Growth factor	Overexpression*	Sarcoma, Glioblastoma
c-hst-1	Growth factor	Overexpression	Stomach, bladder, breast, melanoma
c-erb-B1	Receptor	Overexpression	Lung
c-erb-B2	Receptor	Amplification**	Breast, ovary, lung, stomach
c-erb-B3	Receptor	Overexpression	Breast
c-ret	Receptor	Mutation***	Multiple endocrine neoplasia IIB
c-met	Receptor	Mutation	Kidney (papillary and hereditary)
c-abl	Signal transduction	Translocation**** (9 to 22)	Chronic myeloid leukemia
c-K-ras	Signal transduction	Mutation	Solid tumours (colon, pancreas)
c-N-ras	Signal transduction	Mutation	Acute leukemias
c-N-myc	DNA transcription factor	Amplification	Nephroblastoma (Wilm's tumour)
			Hepatoblastoma
			Small cell lung carcinoma
c-L-myc	DNA transcription factor	Amplification	Small cell lung carcinoma
c-myc	DNA transcription factor	Translocation (8 to 14)	Burkitt's lymphoma

*   Increased expression of protein product
**   Multiplication of genetic sequences
***   Alteration of DNA sequence
****   Exchange of chromosomal material

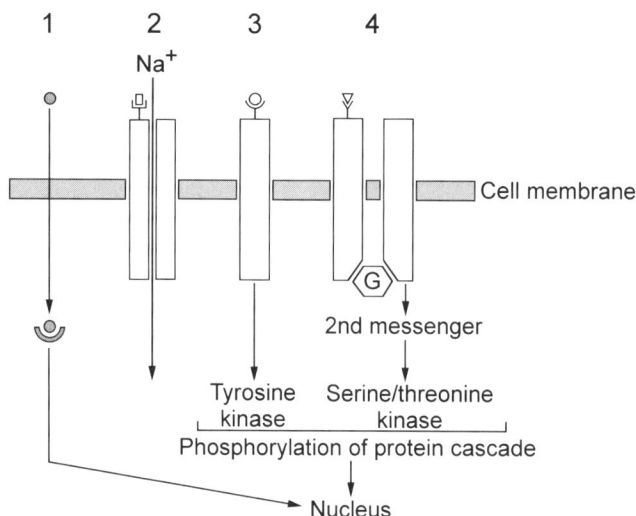

Figure 18 Four principal receptor types involved in signal transduction. 1: cytoplasmic/nuclear receptors for steroid and thyroid hormones. 2: Ion channel in which the ligand may be a neurotransmitter. 3: tyrosine kinase receptor. Ligands include epidermal growth factor, platelet derived growth factor and many other growth factors. 4: G-protein linked receptor. G-proteins belong to a 'superfamily' of related molecules that include the *ras* family of proto-oncogenes. A G-protein (GTP binding protein) stimulates an adjacent enzyme (e.g. adenylate cyclase) which generates cyclic AMP from ATP. This initiates a cascade of protein phosphorylation through serine/threonine kinases. G-proteins may also stimulate cell membrane phosphodiesterases (see page 71).

antibodies. This approach has been utilised in tumour grading and for estimating the size of the proliferative compartment of normal and neoplastic tissues. Flow cytometry provides an automated approach to measuring DNA content, so displaying the cell cycle as a histogram (Fig. 19).

APOPTOSIS

Cell birth must be matched by cell death in order for an organ to remain the same size (Kerr & Searle, 1972). Cell death that occurs under physiological circumstances is the result of an active process that matches the complexity of cell division. It is known as apoptosis, a word used by Homer to describe the dropping off of leaves from autumn trees (Kerr et al., 1972). Apoptosis occurs in normal labile tissues and is also critical in shaping tissues during embryological development (Gräper, 1914). Immune cells that recognise self-antigens are deleted by apoptosis before they can cause self-injury. Cells that are infected by viruses or genetically damaged are removed by apoptosis. Therefore, apoptosis operates under pathological as well as physiological circumstances. The dividing line between apoptosis and necrosis is not absolute, and shared biochemical pathways are now being demonstrated in experimental models of apoptosis and necrosis. For example, the generation of reactive oxygen species appears to characterise *p53*-induced apoptosis as well as hypoxic cell death (Polyak et al., 1997).

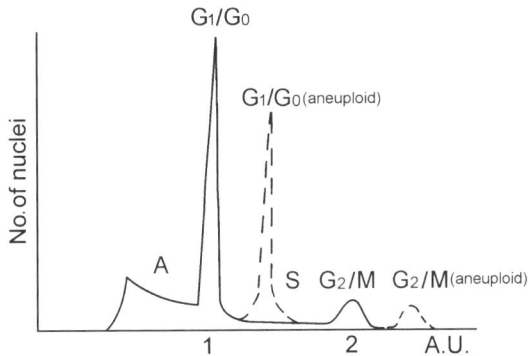

Figure 19 Cell cycle expressed as a flow cytometric histogram. A: Apoptotic cells. A.U.: Arbitrary units of fluorescence. Note the G_2/M peak is exactly double the G_1/G_0 peak, indicating a doubling of DNA content (since the level of fluorescence is directly proportional to DNA content). A second aneuploid population is shown with an abnormal DNA content (dotted line).

The apoptotic cell becomes detached from its normal neighbours to form a round cytoplasmic mass. The cytoplasm is usually deeply eosinophilic, and condensed nuclear material may be present or absent. Phase contrast microscopy of isolated apoptotic cells in culture shows that the cell membrane is thrown into writhing protuberances. These break off to form membrane-bound apoptotic bodies that are only visible at the light microscopic level if they contain basophilic nuclear fragments. Unlike necrosis, apoptosis is not accompanied by an inflammatory reaction. Apoptotic bodies are phagocytosed by adjacent cells or macrophages with great rapidity and are therefore relatively inconspicuous histologically.

A characteristic biochemical change in apoptosis is the cleavage of DNA at regular internucleosomal sites (page 63) by an endonuclease enzyme that is activated by a proteolytic (caspase) cascade (Wyllie, 1980). Apoptosis is regulated by a number of genes and therefore occurs as a result of active gene transcription. Since apoptosis is seen in a variety of physiological and pathological conditions and the decision to die is not taken lightly, even by a cell, the underlying control mechanisms must necessarily be complex. The *p53* tumour suppressor gene is particularly intriguing in this regard. When DNA is damaged by ionising radiation, a decision has to be made to repair the damage if it is slight, or to signal apoptosis if it is severe. In the former case, *p53* signals G_1 arrest to allow time for DNA repair. In the latter case *p53* signals the apoptotic pathway. Since cancer is caused by genetic change it is clear why *p53* is an important tumour suppressor gene (Hooper, 1994). The absence of *p53* will result in genetically altered cells being neither repaired nor deleted.

The therapeutic effects of radiotherapy and chemotherapy are mediated through apoptosis, at least in part, and depend on functioning *p53*. Cancers lacking *p53* are resistant to such treatment (Lowe et al., 1993). *BAX* is another pro-apoptotic tumour suppressor gene, whereas *bcl-2* inhibits apoptosis by stabilising mitochondrial membranes and serves as an oncogene. Cytotoxic T lymphocytes and natural killer cells initiate apoptosis in target cells by engaging with a cell membrane receptor called *fas*. Apoptotic cell death mediated in this way is seen in virus-infected cells, cancer cells, transplant rejection, graft versus host disease and autoimmune diseases (Cummings et al., 1997). It is interesting to note the key involvement of anatomical pathologists not only in the recognition, naming and description of apoptosis, but in appreciating its role in the regulation of growth and development and in disease states (Gräper, 1914; Kerr et al., 1972).

DIFFERENTIATION

Differentiation is more complex and therefore less understood than either mitogenesis or apoptosis. The latter are clear-cut end points for cell populations engaged in turnover. Differentiation encompasses the generation of specialised cells, the organisation of cells into specialised tissues and the processes integrating form and function during embryological development and throughout adult life. Whereas the fundamental mechanisms underlying growth can be explained on the basis of molecular signalling pathways, differentiation involves the control of cell and tissue development as well as molecular transport. Cell to same cell (homotypic), cell to different cell (heterotypic) as well as cell to extracellular matrix interactions must be considered.

Hormones and the more recently investigated retinoids are important mediators of differentiation and development (as well as growth), and the mechanism underlying gene induction by these compounds is now a major research interest. In this section, only the structural basis of cell and tissue differentiation will be reviewed. Interestingly, but consistent with the economy that is so often encountered in nature, there are numerous examples of homologies between the molecular structures underlying the control of growth and differentiation. The cell adhesion molecules, which are introduced below, share structural features with the cell surface receptors that interact with growth factors. Like the growth factor receptors, adhesion molecules have an extracellular domain, a transmembrane domain and an intracellular domain. The intracellular domain may even participate in growth signal transduction. However, the intracellular domain also interacts (through communicating molecules) with a system of microtubules and cytoskeletal filaments. The microtubules are involved in intracellular transport and in mitosis. The cytoskeletal filaments provide a cell with its shape, determine extracellular relationships and participate in various chemo-mechanical activities such as movement, contraction and phagocytosis. The thin filament actin is found in all muscle cells and many other cell types. The thick filament myosin is found in skeletal and cardiac muscle. The family of cell type-specific intermediate-sized filaments includes: cytokeratin (epithelial cells), vimentin (connective tissue cells), desmin (smooth muscle cells), glial fibrillary acid protein (GFAP) (glial cells of the central nervous system), neurofilaments (neurons) and nuclear lamin (nuclei). Monoclonal antibodies raised against the intermediate filaments have proved to be of considerable value in the typing of poorly differentiated cancers (see Chapter 22).

The adhesive molecules are of four main types:

1. Cadherins (E-, N- and P-)

These are Ca^{2+} dependent adhesive molecules involved in homotypic cell to cell interaction. E-cadherin occurs at the junctional complexes (adherens) along the lateral membranes of columnar or cuboidal cells. Loss of the molecule by inherited mutation, acquired mutation (Guildford et al., 1998) or hypermethylation is associated with the development of discohesive signet ring cell carcinoma of the stomach, for example. Signet ring cells are mucus-filled malignant cells and derive their name from the peripherally located nucleus (Fig. 20). N- and P-cadherin are involved in neural cell and placental cell adhesion respectively.

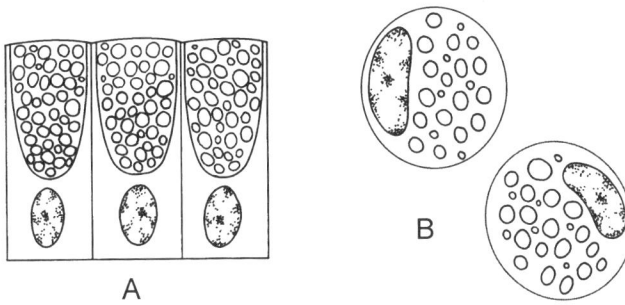

Figure 20 A: Normal columnar mucous cells. B: Discohesive malignant signet ring cells

2. Immunoglobulin-like superfamily

This family includes ICAM-1, ICAM-2, VCAM, and MHC antigens (see Chapter 14). These adhesion molecules are involved in interactions between leukocytes and other cell types. They show structural homologies with immunoglobulins (antibodies), indicating a complex evolutionary relationship for the members of this large family of molecules.

3. Selectins

These transmembrane glycoproteins bind to cell surface antigens expressing carbohydrate structures. Malignant cells in the blood stream may adhere to endothelial cells via E-selectin, a critical step in the metastatic cascade (Chapter 24).

4. Integrins

This family of adhesion molecules is involved in the calcium-dependent binding of cells to matrix proteins and cell to cell (heterotypic) interactions. Anomalous integrin expression is associated with the development of the disturbed growth characteristics of malignant cells (Weaver et al., 1997; Juliano, 1996).

DISORDERS OF GROWTH

Cancer and related disorders are considered in Part IV, though some pertinent points have been referred to in preceding sections of this chapter. Major developmental disorders are described in Chapter 28. Here we consider only hyperplasia, hypertrophy, atrophy and metaplasia (Fig. 21).

Hyperplasia

Hyperplasia refers to an increase in the number of cells in an organ or tissue. It occurs in response to hormonal stimulation, increased functional demand, an abnormal trophic influence or chronic injury. The enlargement of the female breast at puberty is a good example of physiological hyperplasia mediated by oestrogen acting upon the duct epithelium. During pregnancy there is further hyperplasia mediated by progesterone acting on the lobuloalveolar epithelium.

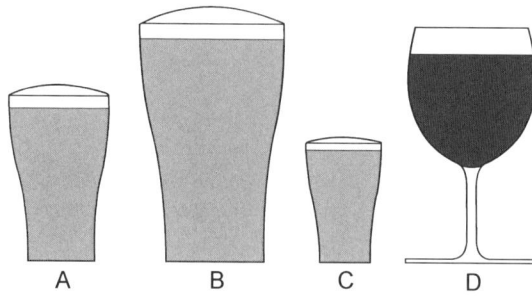

Figure 21 Disorders of growth at the cellular level: normal (A), hypertrophy (B), atrophy (C), metaplasia from columnar cell to goblet cell (D).

Examples of increased functional demand include the hyperplasia of bone marrow (red blood cell precursors) that occurs at high altitude and the enlargement of the parathyroid glands in response to hypocalcemia. Abnormal trophic influences include auto-antibodies directed towards TSH receptors, which cause primary thyrotoxicosis and uncontrolled hormone production by neoplasms (for example bone marrow hyperplasia caused by the secretion of erythropoietin by renal cancers). Chronic irritation and inflammation is a common cause of epithelial hyperplasia in such sites as the gastrointestinal tract, skin and bladder. The mitogenic factors are derived from activated inflammatory cells (T lymphocytes and macrophages) associated with such conditions as chronic gastritis, ulcerative colitis and chronic dermatitis. Hyperplasia is often viewed as a precursor to neoplasia, however the increase in relative risk (presumably related to a slight expansion of the proliferative compartment) varies with the underlying condition and is never marked for the individual patient.

Hypertrophy

Hypertrophy means an increase in the size of a cell. It also describes the increase in size of an organ or tissue, which could be due to cellular hypertrophy, hyperplasia or a combination of the two. Hormonally sensitive tissues show cellular hypertrophy as well as hyperplasia. Prolactin causes enlargement of alveolar epithelial cells in the lactating breast, for example. Permanent tissues such as skeletal and cardiac muscle can only increase in mass by an increase in cell size. The latter occurs in response to exercise or, in the case of the heart, as a consequence of systemic hypertension, outflow obstruction or as a compensatory measure following myocardial infarction. The compensatory enlargement of the remaining kidney following surgical removal of its partner is mainly due to hypertrophy of renal tubular epithelial cells. Cellular hypertrophy is accompanied by an increase in cell function and is mediated by genes involved in signal transduction, including *c-myc, fos, sis* and *ras*.

Atrophy

Atrophy refers to an acquired reduction in cell size and is also used to indicate the size reduction of an organ. The latter is mainly the result of cell loss but remaining cells may be reduced in size. Atrophy may be caused by disease, an inadequate supply of nutrients or oxygen, loss of trophic signals (hormones or growth factors), chronic cell injury (resulting mainly in cell loss) or ageing. Atrophy can be reversed by restoring the missing factors, indicating that atrophy is a form of adaptation that is under genetic control.

Metaplasia

This is the replacement of one differentiated cell type by another. It is seen in situations of chronic inflammation: squamous metaplasia in the respiratory tract in response to tobacco smoke, intestinal metaplasia of the stomach in chronic gastritis, columnar metaplasia of the lower oesophagus in gastro-oesophageal reflux and glandular metaplasia of the chronically inflamed urinary bladder. The extent to which metaplasia is an adaptive phenomenon as opposed to an error in developmental programming is unclear. There is evidence that metaplasia may regress, at least partially, when the causative agent is removed but the change is also associated with an increased risk of cancer. The high frequency and reversibility of metaplasia suggests that genetic mutation is unlikely to be a factor in its aetiology. Epigenetic inactivation of genes, for example by hypermethylation, could explain metaplasia, however.

REFERENCES

Cahill, D.P., Lengauer, C., Yu, J., Riggins, G.J., Willson, J.K.V., Markowitz, S.D., Kinzler, K.W. & Vogelstein, B. (1998) Mutations of mitotic checkpoint genes in human cancers. *Nature,* **392**, 300–303.

Cummings, M.C., Winterford, C.M. & Walker, N.I. (1997) Apoptosis. *Am J Surg Pathol,* **21**, 88–101.

Gräper, L. (1914) Eine neue Anschaung über physiologische Zellausschaltung. Arch Zellforsch, **12**, 373–394.

Guildford, P., Hopkins, J., Harraway, J., McLeod, M., McLeod, N., Harawira, P., Taite, H., Scoular, R., Miller, A. & Reeve, A.E. (1998) E-cadherin germline mutations in familial gastric cancer. *Nature,* **392** 402–405.

Hooper, M.L. (1994) The role of *p53* and *Rb-1* genes in cancer, development and apoptosis. *J Cell Sci*, **18**, 13–17.

Juliano, R. (1996) Cooperation between soluble factors and integrin-mediated cell anchorage in the control of growth and differentiation. *Bioassays,* **18**, 911–917.

Kaufman, W.K. & Paules, R.S. (1996) DNA damage and cell cycle checkpoints. *FASEB J,* **10**, 238–247.

Kerr, J.F.R., Wyllie, A.M. & Currie, A.R. (1972) Apoptosis: a basic biological phenomenon with wide-ranging implications in tissue kinetics. *Br J Cancer,* **26**, 239–257.

Kerr, J.F.R. & Searle, J. (1972) A suggested explanation for the paradoxically slow growth rate of basal-cell carcinomas that contain numerous apoptotic figures. *J Pathol,* **107**, 41–44.

Lowe, S.W., Ruley, H.E., Jacks, T. & Housman, D.E. (1993) p53-dependent apoptosis modulates the cytotoxicity of anticancer agents. *Cell,* **74**, 957–967.

Polyak, K., Xia, Y., Zweiter, J.L., Kinzler, K.W. & Vogelstein, B. (1997) A model for p53 induced apoptosis. *Nature,* **389**, 300–305.

Weaver, V.M., Peterson, O.W., Wang, F., Larabell, C.A., Briand, P., Damsky, C. & Bissell, M.J. (1997) Reversion of the malignant phenotype of human breast cells in three dimensional culture and *in vivo* by integrin blocking antibodies. *J Cell Biol*, **137**, 231–245.

Wyllie, A.H. (1980) Glucocorticoid-induced thymocyte apoptosis is associated with endogenous endonuclease activation. *Nature*, **284**, 555–556.

Further reading

Berry, C.L. (1995) The molecular basis of development. In *Progress in Pathology*, volume 1, edited by N. Kirkham & P. Hall, pp. 121–132. Edinburgh: Churchill Livingstone,

Pezzella, F. & Gatter, K. (1995) What is the value of bcl-2 protein detection for histopathologists? *Histopathology*, **26**, 89–93.

Pignatelli, M. & Vessey, C.J. (1995) Adhesion molecules and cancer. In *Progress in Pathology*, Volume 2, edited by Kirkham, N. & Lemoine, N.R., pp. 159–175. Edinburgh: Churchill Livingstone.

Potten, C.S. (1987) *Perspectives on Mammalian Cell Death*. Oxford: Oxford University Press.

Wyllie, A.H. (1997) Apoptosis. In *Recent Advances in Histopathology*, volume 17, edited by P.P. Anthony, R.N.M. MacSween & D.G. Lowe, pp. 1–14. Edinburgh: Churchill Livingstone.

— PART III —

BLOOD, TUBES, FLUIDS AND FLOW

17

OEDEMA, HAEMORRHAGE
AND THROMBOSIS

*Nature is nowhere accustomed more openly to display her secret mysteries
than in cases where she shows traces of her workings apart from the beaten
path; nor is there any better way to advance the proper practice of medicine
than to give our minds to the discovery of the usual law of Nature by careful
investigation of cases of rare forms of disease*

William Harvey, 1657

How do bruises come and go?

HISTORICAL PERSPECTIVES ON THE CIRCULATION

The natural philosophers of ancient Greece believed that 'pneuma' (roughly equivalent to
spirit or air) was endowed with the properties of life and intelligence. While the balance of the
four humours determined the state of health and temperament of an individual, pneuma was
the source of thought and sensation. Erasistratus (310–250 BC) of Ceos, known as the father
of physiology, recognised the circulation of blood through the veins and right ventricle of
the heart, but believed that pneuma flowed from the lungs to the left ventricle and then to the
rest of the body via the arterial system. Ironically, the occurrence of blood within the arterial
system was deemed pathological. Galen believed that the brain was the seat of the mind and
appreciated the role of the blood in the support and nutrition of the fabric of the body. He
showed that arteries pumped bright red blood (by ligating and opening an arterial segment in
a living animal), but still believed that the two sides of the circulation were unconnected. He
reasoned that blood was enriched with nutrition from the gut and then flowed to the liver
(where it was purified). This fits well with modern thinking. However upon ebbing into the
right side of the heart, Galen believed, it then flowed straight back out again (as a tidal motion)
via the veins to give nutrition to all parts of the body including the lungs. Galen explained his
demonstration of blood in the arterial system by the presence of invisible 'pores' in the
septum of the heart (Jackson, 1988).

The anatomist Andreas Vesalius (1514–1564) did not accept Galens's pores, but it is William
Harvey (1578–1657) who is credited with the modern explanation of blood circulation.

However, Harvey believed that the arteries ended blindly in the tissues, like spring water lost in the sand, to be gathered up by the veins, like underground water returning to a rivulet. With the aid of living frogs and a microscope, Marcello Malpighi (1628–1694) discovered the microcirculation and so proved that the blood flow in the dual circulation was not only one-way, but continuous and uninterrupted (Doby, 1963). The concept of 'pneuma' still persists today through such terms as prana (Sanskrit), life force (elan vital) and life blood. Whilst these terms have no scientific validity, it is certainly true that cardiovascular disease is today the leading cause of morbidity and death within the industrialised nations. The susceptibility of the cardiovascular system and specifically the heart to life-threatening disease was presaged as recently as 1876 when Adam Hammer, Professor of Surgery at St Louis, Missouri, was called to the bedside of a 34-year-old man who had collapsed suddenly and become cyanosed with a slowed pulse. Virchow had earlier described venous thrombosis and listed the three predisposing factors: abnormal turbulence, damage to the vein wall and increased stickiness of the blood (Virchow's triad). Hammer diagnosed thrombotic occlusion of at least one coronary artery. This was confirmed at autopsy and reported as the first case of coronary thrombosis in the Viennese Medical Journal in 1878 (Major, 1978).

James Herrick, Professor of Medicine in Chicago from 1900, correlated the clinical features of sudden coronary artery occlusion with autopsy findings in the Journal of the American Medical Association in 1912. In retrospect, it seems remarkable that such a common condition was not fully documented until well into the twentieth century (White, 1974).

OEDEMA

Water comprises about 60% of the lean body weight, a little more than half of which is intracellular, the remainder being extracellular. The latter is found within the plasma of the bloodstream (20%) and in the spaces surrounding cells (interstitium) (80%). Only very small amounts of fluid are found within body cavities (pericardium, pleural, peritoneal, and joint cavities). Exceptions are the ventricular system and subarachnoid space of the central nervous system and the chambers of the eye. Given our watery nature, it is not surprising that the circulation and body fluids feature so prominently in medical practice.

Oedema describes the abnormal collection of fluid within the extracellular compartment. Such collections will occur within the body cavities (as effusions in the pleural and pericardial cavities or ascites in the peritoneal cavity), within loose and relatively acellular connective tissue (dermis of skin, subcutaneous tissue or submucosa of gut), within the brain or within the alveolar spaces of the lungs. These accumulations are derived from the blood and are formed on the basis of four mechanisms:

1. Acute inflammation associated with a leaky microvasculature, when the fluid will be a protein rich exudate.

2. Increased hydrostatic pressure. Common causes are right heart failure (congestive cardiac failure) and venous thrombosis. The former causes bilateral lower limb oedema which 'pits' when finger pressure is applied; latter causes a localised oedema.

3. Reduced plasma osmotic pressure due to a reduction in the concentration of large osmotically active molecules (proteins such as albumin) that do not normally leave the bloodstream. This may be due to abnormal loss of protein in the urine (nephrotic syndrome), cirrhosis of the liver (the main source of synthesis of plasma proteins) or severe protein malnutrition.

4.   Obstruction of lymphatic vessels whose function is to drain fluid from interstitial spaces and return it to the circulation. Causes may be invasion of lymphatic vessels by cancer, worm larvae (causing elephantiasis), surgical transection (for example dissection of axillary lymph nodes for breast cancer causing oedema of the upper limb) and damage to lymphatics caused by radiotherapy.

When the cause of oedema is heart failure or reduced plasma osmotic pressure, the contracted plasma volume results in reduced kidney perfusion. In response to this, the kidney secretes renin which activates plasma angiotensin which in turn acts upon the adrenal cortex to cause release of the hormone aldosterone. Aldosterone promotes sodium (and water) reabsorption from the distal tubules of the renal nephrons (in exchange for potassium). This increases the fluid load and therefore hydrostatic pressure, but there will be worsening of the oedema. Because of the redistribution of sodium-rich fluid as oedema, blood sodium levels may be low even though the total body sodium is increased. The patient needs to lose sodium and water and, as recorded by the nineteenth century physician William Osler, congestive cardiac failure was one disease that was actually improved by the ancient art of blood-letting. Diuretic drugs are used for the same purpose in the modern era, but blood letting (venesection) is still used to treat haemochromatosis (an inherited autosomal recessive disorder causing iron overload and cirrhosis of the liver) and polycythemia (a bone marrow disorder resulting in excess production of red blood cells).

TRANSUDATES AND EXUDATES

When swollen oedematous tissue is viewed microscopically, one sees only a widening of the clear space between cells. Pink (eosinophilic) staining is caused by the presence of protein and the polymer fibrin formed by coagulation (see below), and reflects an effusion that is particularly high in protein. This is called an exudate and occurs in a background of acute inflammation. Oedema fluid caused by the remaining mechanisms is protein-poor and is called a transudate. Acute pulmonary oedema caused by left heart failure is easily visualised macroscopically (at autopsy) because the lungs are heavy and appear like fluid-filled sponges. Microscopically, pulmonary oedema may be overlooked when the protein concentration is low and the alveoli are filled with inconspicuous, very pale pink, finely granular material.

HYPERAEMIA AND CONGESTION

An increased volume of blood within an organ is described as active hyperaemia (or just hyperaemia) when it is caused by increased arterial blood flow, as in acute inflammation or blushing, or congestion (passive hyperaemia) when the cause is reduced venous outflow. Both hyperaemia and congestion are associated with oedema.

Pulmonary congestion and oedema is caused by left heart failure, but is most marked when there is stenosis (narrowing) of the mitral valve resulting in compensatory work hypertrophy of the muscular wall of the left atrium. This in turn leads to a substantial increase in pressure within the left atrium that is transmitted back to the pulmonary microvasculature via the pulmonary veins. The delicate capillaries within the septal walls of the alveoli will rupture, allowing red blood cells to escape into the interstitial spaces and the alveoli. Alveolar macrophages engulf the red blood cell debris and the haemoglobin is broken down to be stored within these 'heart failure cells' as the brown iron-containing pigment haemosiderin (see haemorrhage below). Sputum coughed up by patients with mitral stenosis may be rust coloured due to the presence of these cells.

Right heart failure leads to congestion within the sinusoids of the liver and spleen. Sinusoids are lined by endothelial cells (like capillaries), but are separated by fenestrations (gaps) and lack a supporting basement membrane, a design that allows cells such as motile phagocytic cells to squeeze in and out of sinusoids with ease. The macroscopic appearance of a congested liver upon slicing has been likened to a section through a nutmeg. The dark fern-like tracery is the blood that has accumulated in the sinusoids and central vein of the microscopic liver lobules. The term 'nutmeg liver' dates back to the autopsy days of Karl Rokitansky.

HAEMORRHAGE

Rupture of a small blood vessel in the skin or membranes of the body may cause pinpoint haemorrhages (petechiae), larger spots (purpura) or still larger bruises (ecchymoses). A large accumulation of blood that is bordered by tissue planes is called a haematoma. Haemorrhage into a body cavity, such as the pericardium following rupture of the heart wall, is termed a haemopericardium.

The interior of a red blood cell consists almost exclusively of the oxygen-carrying molecule haemoglobin. Following haemorrhage, the red blood cell lyses, releasing haemoglobin, and the cellular debris is phagocytosed by macrophages. Haemoglobin splits into the haem (the oxygen-carrying part of haemoglobin) and the protein globin. (Haem, derived from ingested blood, is readily absorbed by the gut and is the main source of dietary iron.) Haem is broken down further into iron and biliverdin. The latter is a green-coloured pigment and this explains why bruises change from blue to green. Bruises become yellow due to the conversion of biliverdin to bilirubin (which translates as 'red bile' but is in fact yellow). Bilirubin is rendered soluble by being bound to albumin. It passes into the circulation from which it is extracted by the liver and conjugated (since albumin is too large to pass through the kidney filter). The excess iron at the site of haemorrhage is taken up and stored within macrophages as golden brown haemosiderin. Macrophages containing haemosiderin (siderophages) may remain at the site of haemorrhage for weeks, months, or years, serving as a microscopic and sometimes macroscopic marker of the earlier event.

BLOOD CLOTTING OR COAGULATION

Bleeding is controlled physiologically by a combination of haemostatic mechanisms: (1) vasoconstriction brought about by the contraction of vascular smooth muscle (controlled by the autonomic nervous system and locally-released chemical mediators), (2) coagulation, and (3) platelet aggregation (thrombosis) (see below).

Clotting or coagulation simply implies the conversion of the soluble plasma protein fibrinogen into the insoluble, jelly-like polymer fibrin. The fibrin so formed assists in the plugging of damaged vessels in association with aggregated platelets (see below). In the context of acute inflammation, fibrin entraps bacteria and therefore prevents their spread and assists in their elimination. Clearly such a process must be regulated carefully otherwise the entire circulation could become blocked with coagulated blood. Something like this in fact happens under certain circumstances and is called disseminated intravascular coagulation (DIC). When this occurs in a mild form relatively small vessels may be blocked in organs such as the kidney. This may not be life-threatening because of the reserve capacity of most organs and the potential for reversal. In severe DIC, the main problem is the massive consumption of the clotting factors, which must be replaced to prevent catastrophic haemorrhage. DIC may be a terminal manifestation of life-threatening disorders such as severe sepsis, meningococcal meningitis, massive tissue injury, advanced adenocarcinoma, leukaemia (acute promyelocytic type), snakebites, and various complications of pregnancy. The underlying mechanism in each case is overactivation of the coagulation pathway coupled with the overwhelming (i.e. relative failure) of the opposing fibrinolytic (fibrin degradation) mechanism predisposing to tissue ischaemia as well as lethal haemorrhage.

Coagulation occurs not only in living organisms, but also postmortem and even within a test tube. In life, the process is initiated by release of 'tissue factor' from damaged tissues and occurs in a series of amplifying steps likened to a cascade. Briefly, a clotting factor in the form of an active enzyme acts upon a substrate converting it in turn into an active enzyme, and so on. Factors VIII (calcium-dependent) and V act outside the cascade, serving as accelerators. There is little point in memorising the order of the cascade, particularly as most of the longer 'intrinsic' cascade does not have an important role in the living organism. The penultimate step involves the conversion of factor II (prothrombin) to thrombin which finally converts fibrinogen to fibrin. The factors are synthesised by the liver, and chronic liver damage (cirrhosis) will result in factor deficiency and therefore a bleeding tendency. Amongst the functioning factors are II, VII, IX and X. The synthesis of these requires the presence of vitamin K. Vitamin K deficiency occurs in association with fat malabsorption (since it is fat soluble and therefore lost in fatty stools) and in neonates (since little crosses the placenta). The sex-linked forms of haemophilia (female carriers and affected males) result in excessive bruising due to deficiency of factor VIII (haemophilia A) and factor IX (haemophilia B or Christmas disease).

A system exists for containing and regulating the clotting cascade. This involves the formation of plasmin from plasminogen, which breaks down fibrin into fibrin-degradation products (fibrinolysis). Multiple factors serve to activate or inhibit the generation of plasmin from plasminogen, thereby fine-tuning the system.

THROMBOSIS

The term thrombosis describes the haemostatic process of platelet aggregation with concurrent formation of fibrin. It is also used to indicate the exaggerated process resulting in the formation of a pathological mass within the bloodstream. Physiological haemostasis and abnormal platelet aggregation differ quantitatively only. Platelets are small, non-nucleated, membrane-bound cytoplasmic fragments found within blood and formed by budding off from large multinucleated cells called megakaryocytes which are located within the bone marrow. They are of fundamental importance in the process of normal haemostasis. Endothelial injury leads to platelet adhesion (by the platelet adhesion molecule P-selectin) and aggregation, particularly upon exposure of the underlying basement membrane collagen. The adherent platelets attract more platelets by secreting ADP, thromboxane A_2 and serotonin. There is simultaneous activation of coagulation upon the platelet membrane which utilises fibrinogen released by the platelet. Additional factors serve to promote platelet aggregation, including thrombin and von Willebrand factor, the latter being released by damaged endothelial cells. Von Willebrand's disease is a bleeding disorder resulting in deficiency of the factor and is inherited as an autosomal dominant trait. Platelet deficiency, affecting either numbers or function, is a further cause of bleeding disorders.

The three major influences that promote abnormal thrombosis are: (1) vascular (endothelial) injury, (2) alteration to blood flow, and (3) hypercoagulability. These comprise Virchow's triad. The particular combination will be influenced by site within the cardiovascular system. Endothelial injury is crucial within the left heart and the fast flowing arterial system. The main causes of endothelial injury will be myocardial infarction leading to mural thrombosis in the left ventricle, infective and non-infective endocarditis of the heart valves (the latter occurring in terminally ill patients with cancer) and atherosclerosis. In the venous system, prolonged pressure on deep calf veins (e.g. during surgery) is likely to cause mild endothelial injury. Alteration to blood flow will occur in an aneurysm of the left ventricle or aorta, a fibrillating left atrium and in the situation of stasis within the deep veins of the leg. Hypercoagulability occurs in a number of clinical settings including severe trauma, cancer, multiple haematological disorders, late pregnancy and during treatment with oral contraceptives. A number of anti-thrombotic factors exist including antithrombin III, protein S and protein C. A deficiency of any of these may occur on an inherited basis leading to an increased risk of thrombosis.

Thrombi formed in the fast-moving arterial system tend to be small, friable, pale and platelet-rich. Those developing within aneurysms (left ventricular or aortic) show well-developed lines of Zahn. These are pale, platelet-rich lines alternating with fibrin-rich lines that contain admixed red blood cells. Those developing in the relatively sluggish venous system (phlebothrombosis) are composed mainly of fibrin and admixed red blood cells but will still be firmer and drier than a postmortem blood clot. Furthermore, small numbers of platelets will be seen microscopically. Postmortem blood clot is soft, jelly-like and is never firmly adherent to the vessel wall in which it forms. It may be composed largely of yellow coagulated plasma, when it has been likened to 'chicken fat'. The distinction is important when trying to decide at a postmortem examination if a mass within the pulmonary artery is embolised thrombus (see Chapter 18) or merely postmortem blood clot.

Thrombosis may be fatal if there is sudden occlusion of a vital vessel such as a coronary artery. If the patient survives, a thrombus may continue to increase in length (propagate), embolise to distant sites (see Chapter 18), dissolve completely or undergo organisation when it is replaced by granulation tissue and finally converted to fibrous tissue showing at least partial recanalisation.

REFERENCES

Doby, T. (1963) *Discoverers of blood circulation. From Aristotle to the times of da Vinci and Harvey*. London: Abelard-Schuman.

Herrick, J.B. (1971) Clinical factors of sudden obstruction of the coronary arteries. *JAMA* 1912, **58**.

Major, R.H. (1978) *Classic Descriptions of Disease* (3rd edn). Springfield, Illinois: Charles C Thomas, pp 424–8.

White, P.D. (1974) The historical background of angina pectoris. *Mod Concepts Cardiovasc Dis*, **18**, 109.

18

EMBOLISM, ISCHAEMIA, INFARCTION AND SHOCK

It is my duty to tell you that death from this disease is often sudden

Lydgate to Casaubon in *Middlemarch* by George Eliot

What events may lead to ischaemic necrosis?

EMBOLISM

Embolism is the passage of a mass (an embolus) within the bloodstream from a point of origin to a point of impaction. The embolus may be a solid, a liquid or a gas. Although the majority of emboli arise from thrombi (see Chapter 17), the importance of the atheromatous plaque as a source of embolic material has been underestimated (Chapter 19). Nevertheless, for the purposes of this chapter, the unqualified use of the term embolism refers to thromboembolism.

Emboli can be classified conveniently into (1) those arising in the deep veins of the lower limb which pass through the right side of the heart to impact within the pulmonary arterial circulation, and (2) systemic emboli arising mainly within the left ventricle, the left atrium, the valves of the left heart or large arteries which impact within the systemic arterial circulation.

Pulmonary embolism

Depending on its size, the embolism may obstruct the main pulmonary trunk, the site of bifurcation of the pulmonary trunk into the right and left pulmonary arteries (saddle embolism), or one or more branches of a pulmonary artery. A massive pulmonary embolism is a cause of sudden death. At autopsy a large embolism is usually noted to be coiled up into an obstructing mass. It is drier and firmer than a blood clot. Although it may be firmly impacted within a vessel, it does not form a perfect cast. Histological examination will confirm the presence of platelet aggregates as well as fibrin.

Most pulmonary emboli produce no clinical symptoms because they are small and the pulmonary reserve is large. Obstruction of a larger branch of a pulmonary artery tends not to produce an area of ischaemic necrosis (infarction). The lung has a dual blood supply: deoxygenated blood via the pulmonary arterial system, and oxygenated blood via the bronchial arteries. The bronchial arterial supply protects pulmonary tissues from ischaemia unless the circulation is compromised by an additional factor such as heart failure. Showers of emboli that become lodged and organised may, if present in sufficient numbers, lead to increased resistance within the pulmonary arterial tree, and so cause pulmonary hypertension. Emboli arising from the deep veins of the leg may only enter the systemic circulation if there is a septal defect in the heart. This is known as paradoxical embolism but is extremely uncommon.

Systemic embolism

A high proportion of systemic emboli arise from a mural thrombus secondary to a myocardial infarct. A mural thrombus is attached to the endocardial side of the infarcted heart wall. Detached fragments may embolise to the lower limbs, brain or organs such as the kidney, gut and spleen. Other sources are an atrial thombus (in a patient with atrial fibrillation), or an infected thrombus from the aortic or mitral valve of a subject with infective endocarditis. Atheromatous embolism is discussed on page 122.

Other types of embolism

Amniotic fluid embolism following childbirth is unpreventable and highly dangerous, though fortunately is very rare. In lethal cases the diagnosis is confirmed at autopsy by the finding of squamous cells and debris of fetal origin impacted within branches of the pulmonary artery.

Air may enter the circulation as a result of therapeutic procedures, but small volumes are not dangerous. Deep sea divers, however, are at risk of air embolism. Inert gases (nitrogen) breathed in under pressure are readily absorbed, but if the diver ascends too rapidly the gases are released as bubbles within the circulation, which obstruct small vessels. The acute form of diving sickness is known as 'the bends' and presents with severe musculoskeletal pain, respiratory distress and, in severe cases, coma leading to death. A chronic form is associated with multiple bone infarcts (Caisson disease).

Fat embolism occurs commonly following the fracture of the shafts of long bones, which contain a fatty marrow, but produces serious symptoms in only a small proportion of subjects with severe trauma.

Foreign bodies, such as bullets, are also occasionally shown to have embolised.

ISCHAEMIA

The term ischaemia refers to a reduction in the blood supply to tissues, and is an important cause of tissue necrosis. An infarct is an area of ischaemic necrosis. The flow of blood through a tissue is cut off in a final and complete way if an end artery is occluded by a thrombus. The thrombus may be embolic or may develop *in situ* on an atheromatous plaque (Chapter 19). Alternatively, an artery may be occluded by external factors, for example, mechanical twisting of a loop of bowel (see Chapter 32). Ischaemia will be partial or relative in tissues receiving a collateral blood supply or a dual blood supply, or if the obstruction is to the venous outflow. Under such circumstances the risk of infarction will be influenced by additional determinants of tissue perfusion such as heart pump efficiency (heart failure), transient hypotension, disease of the tissue in question (left ventricular hypertrophy), or partial narrowing of the arteries or arterioles supplying the tissue. In other words, ischaemic necrosis may occur without complete arterial occlusion.

INFARCTION

Infarction is the process of circumscribed tissue necrosis brought about through ischaemia. The main mechanisms are presented in the preceding section. Infarcts are either pale or red. Pale infarcts occur in solid organs such as the heart, spleen or kidney, and always come about through arterial occlusion. Initially there may be haemorrhage as a result of collateral blood flow, but the red blood cells eventually lyse and the infarct becomes increasingly pale. Red infarcts occur in tissues with a dual blood supply (lung) or a rich system of collateral vessels (gut). Venous occlusion does not usually result in infarction, but when it does the infarcts are red. Cerebral infarcts may be red as a result of secondary haemorrhage caused by restored blood flow into tissues containing damaged vessels.

Regardless of colour, infarcts are approximately wedge-shaped with the apex of the wedge at the site of arterial occlusion and the base at the external edge of the affected organ. This reflects the fact that an artery will divide and fan out beyond the blockage to supply a wedge-shaped zone of tissue (cone shaped in three dimensions). Necrosis is a cause of inflammation, and a red zone composed of reactive granulation tissue is seen at the periphery of a sectioned pale infarct that is a few days old (Fig. 22). Histologically, all infacts, apart from those in the brain, show coagulative necrosis. The dead tissue is digested and phagocytosed by macrophages and replaced (organised) by granulation tissue which ultimately forms a dense scar. In the brain there is liquefactive necrosis, and the infarcted zone is converted into a cystic space after the debris has been removed by macrophages (derived from microglia).

SHOCK

The term shock refers to a state of circulatory collapse resulting in generalised hypoperfusion of tissues and hypotension when compensatory mechanisms break down. The least

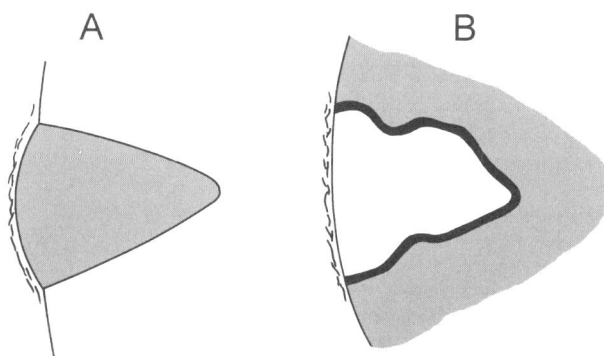

Figure 22 A: Red infarct of lung with bulging pleural surface covered with a fibrinous exudate. B: Pale infarct of myocardium with a rim of inflamed granulation tissue and an overlying fibrinous pericarditis.

dangerous form of shock is vasovagal shock or fainting. Anaphylactic shock is a result of severe generalised type I hypersensitivity, in which massive histamine release leads to widespread vasodilation (treated by administration of adrenaline). The most common and clinically important forms of shock are: (1) cardiogenic shock due to sudden failure of the myocardial pump, (2) hypovolaemic shock due to acute loss of blood or body fluids, and (3) septic shock due to the intravascular spread of bacteria from sites of local infection.

In a state of shock the organs at greatest risk are the brain, heart, lungs, kidneys, gut and adrenals. If the patient survives, ischaemic loss of neurons and myocardial cells is irreversible. The kidney is susceptible to the development of acute tubular necrosis which presents with renal failure, however, regeneration of renal tubules may occur with complete recovery of renal function. Shock caused by bacterial sepsis or severe trauma may result in diffuse alveolar damage of the lungs, a condition known as shock lung or adult respiratory distress syndrome (ARDS). The alveolus becomes lined with a hyaline (amorphous pink) membrane composed of fibrin which interferes with gaseous exchange. If the patient survives, the fibrin may either be removed or organised into fibrous tissue, which may lead to the development of 'honeycomb lung' (page 214). The adrenals show a characteristic shock sequence in which the yellow lipid of the cortical cells is converted into steroid hormones and therefore disappears.

Septic shock is a common cause of death in intensive therapy units and amongst elderly subjects, in whom the symptoms and signs of infection are often attenuated and therefore easily overlooked. Autopsy examination shows that both infection and septic shock are underdiagnosed, particularly in the elderly. The primary sources of infection may be abscesses, peritonitis, pneumonia, infective endocarditis or urinary tract infections. Gram negative bacilli such as *Escherichia coli*, *Klebsiella pneumoniae*, *Proteus* species, *Bacteroides* species and *Pseudomonas aeruginosa* produce an endotoxin (a bacterial wall liposaccharide) which triggers the shock response. Septic shock may also be caused by toxins generated by gram positive cocci (toxic shock syndrome).

Septic shock results when the bacterially derived endotoxin ligand binds to receptors on inflammatory cells and endothelial cells. This results in the uncontrolled release of inflammatory mediators, resulting in turn in direct tissue damage, circulatory collapse and disseminated intravascular coagulation. All inflammatory mediators have been implicated in septic shock, including cytokines (IL-1 and tumour necrosis factor-α), platelet activating factor and nitric oxide (Parrillo, 1993).

REFERENCES

Parrillo, J.E. (1993) Pathogenetic mechanisms of septic shock. *N Engl J Med,* **328**, 1471–1477.

Further reading

Krausz, T. & Cohen, J. (1992) Shock. In *Oxford Textbook of Pathology,* edited by J. O'D, McGee, P.G. Isaacson & N.A. Wright, pp. 540–541. Oxford: Oxford University Press.

Woolf, N.A. (1992) Embolism. In *Oxford Textbook of Pathology,* edited by J. O'D, McGee, P.G. Isaacson & N.A. Wright, pp. 521–524. Oxford: Oxford University Press.

Woolf, N.A. (1992) Ischaemia and infarction. In *Oxford Textbook of Pathology,* edited by J. O'D, McGee, P.G. Isaacson & N.A. Wright, pp. 524–530. Oxford: Oxford University Press.

19

ATHEROSCLEROSIS, ARTERIOLOSCLEROSIS AND VASCULITIS

So far no-one has brought to light anything valid
concerning the connections between veins and arteries

Marcello Malpighi (1628–1694)

What type of disorder is atherosclerosis?

ENDOTHELIAL CELLS AND INTIMA

Common to all the vessels of the body—arteries, arterioles, capillaries, venules, veins and lymphatics— is a central channel or lumen bounded by flattened endothelial cells forming a sheet known as endothelium. Endothelial cells may be separated by spaces in the case of specialised capillaries such as sinusoids in the liver. The endothelial cells, like all cells lining a surface, rest upon a continuous basement membrane. In larger vessels the endothelium is supported by a thin connective tissue layer which together comprise the innermost vascular layer known as the intima. Outside the intima, and particularly well-developed in arteries, is a concentric layer of smooth muscle called the media, and outside this is a third layer formed of connective tissue called the adventitia. The media of arteries is bounded internally and externally by a distinct lamina (sheet) of elastin.

Endothelial cells form the interface between the flow of blood and the rest of the body and are therefore required to be both tough and versatile. They respond rapidly to many chemical mediators of acute inflammation (see Chapter 12), and express a variety of adhesion molecules upon their surface membranes when so induced (by cytokines elaborated by monocytes and lymphocytes). Endothelial cells also orchestrate the process of thrombosis (see Chapter 17) in response to both physiological and pathological stimuli.

ATHEROSCLEROSIS

Atherosclerosis, the scourge of the Western world, is essentially a disease of the intima of larger arteries, particularly those supplying the heart and brain, as well as the abdominal aorta. The spectrum of intimal thickening ranges from normal adaptive thickening present at birth, early lesions (types I and II or fatty streak), preatheroma (type III) and advanced raised lesions (types IV–VIII) (Stary, 1996).

The atheromatus plaque of the advanced lesion consists of a fibrous roof (consisting of collagen synthesised by the modified smooth muscle cells) overlying atheroma, a soft, yellow centre composed of necrotic material and lipid lying free as cholesterol crystals or within foamy macrophages (Fig. 23) (Woolf, 1990). (The word atheroma means gruel or porridge in Greek and describes the soft yellow sludge.) The interest of the atheromatous plaque lies in the seriousness of its complications and in its causation. Knowledge of the causation might lead to the introduction of preventive strategies that would have a major impact upon morbidity and death in the Western world.

Complications

As the atheromatous plaque increases in size, it may undergo dystrophic calcification and cause progressive narrowing of the lumen of the artery. Complete and sudden occlusion may be caused by haemorrhage into the necrotic interior of the plaque, thereby lifting it up. Alternatively, occlusion may be caused by thrombosis on the surface of an ulcerated plaque. Severe atherosclerosis of the aorta may be associated with extensive plaque ulceration with exposure of the soft, crumbly interior. The latter may be swept away within the bloodstream to produce atheroembolism.

In addition to larger atheromatous particles—which may occlude small arteries in the kidney, gut or skin of lower limb causing ischaemic injury—is the more common phenomenon of cholesterol crystal embolisation (Moolenaar & Lamers, 1996). Groups of crystals will occlude arterioles, and if showers of crystals are being released continuously, ischaemic damage will eventuate (again mainly in the kidney, gut and skin of lower limb). Gut involvement usually presents with bleeding, the source of which may be difficult to determine. At autopsy, cholesterol crystal embolism is surprisingly common (3–18%). The crystals appear as a row of slits (the enclosed crystals are dissolved out during the preparation of the slide) partly surrounded by foreign body multinucleate giant cells and eosinophils.

Severe atheroma may also weaken the wall of an artery, causing it to dilate and form an aneurysm (Fig. 24). Aneurysms may rupture, causing catastrophic haemorrhage. Key factors in the pathogenesis of all aneurysms are mural weakening and/or systemic hypertension.

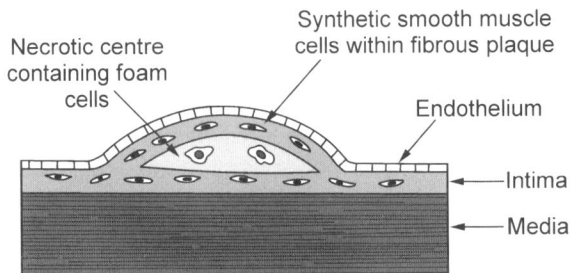

Figure 23 Structure of an atheromatous plaque

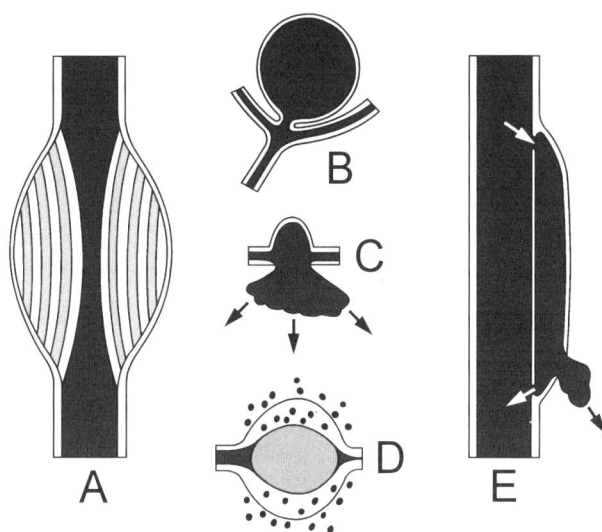

Figure 24 Types of arterial aneurysm. A: A fusiform aneurysm of the abdominal aorta, a complication of severe atherosclerosis. Laminated thrombus (lines of Zahn formed of platelets and red blood cells entrapped in fibrin) fills the aneurysm and narrows the lumen. The weakened wall may rupture. B: A berry aneurysm occurring at a site of bifurcation in the circle of Willis. This may rupture causing haemorrhage into the subarachnoid space. C: A ruptured micro-aneurysm of a small intracerebral artery is the major cause of haemorrhagic stroke (cerebrovascular accident). D: Aneurysm caused by inflammatory weakening of the arterial wall. This may be caused by lodgment of a bacterially infected thromboembolism (mycotic aneurysm) or a hypersensitivity arteritis caused by circulating immune complexes. Mycotic aneurysms are more destructive and cause rupture and haemorrhage. Arteritis is associated with occlusive thrombosis and distal ischaemic injury. E: Dissecting aneurysm (typically in thoracic aorta) in which blood enters a weakened media through an intimal tear. Blood may rupture back into the lumen to form a double-barrelled aorta or outwards causing a lethal haemorrhage.

Causes and pathogenesis

Epidemiological studies have shown that the major risk factors of atherosclerosis are diet (i.e. one high in cholesterol), hyperlipidemia of genetic origin, hypertension, smoking and diabetes mellitus. Other risk factors include male gender, obesity, age and physical inactivity. In the past, two main theories were put forward to explain the growth of an atheromatous plaque. The first envisaged the insudation of cholesterol from the bloodstream into the intima, this in turn stimulating the proliferation of smooth muscle cells. The second theory focused on the progressive laying down and organisation of platelet thrombi. The contemporary view combines elements of both theories but views atherosclerosis as an inflammatory response to intimal injury (Ross & Fuster, 1996). The suggested steps are shown in Figure 25. Thrombosis is now viewed as a late complication of atheroma, rather than as a predisposing event. The sequence of events outlined in Figure 25 fits with the risk posed by hypercholesterolemia and the direct damaging influence of hypertension and cigarette smoke upon endothelial cells.

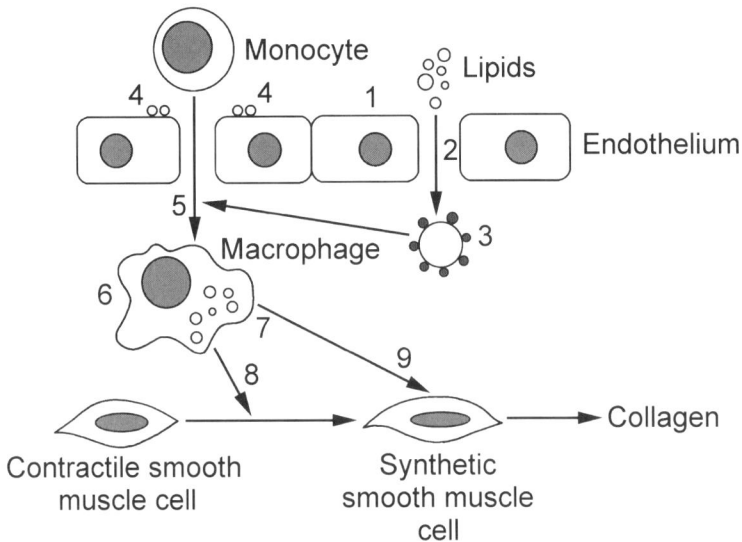

Figure 25 Steps in the pathogenesis of atherosclerosis are as follows: 1. Endothelial cell dysfunction; 2. Increased permeability to plasma lipids; 3. Oxidation of plasma lipids by endothelial cells, smooth muscle cells and macrophages; 4. Adhesion of monocytes and platelets to endothelium; 5. Migration of monocytes into intima under chemotaxic influence of oxidized plasma lipids; 6. Transformation of monocytes into macrophages; 7. Phagocytosis of lipid by macrophages which become foam cells; 8. Macrophages degrade basement membrane matrix of contractile smooth muscle cells which migrate into intima to become synthetic smooth muscle cells; 9. Growth factors synthesized by macrophages (PDGF and TGFβ) promote division of synthetic smooth muscle cells and collagen production (Campbell & Campbell, 1994).

Considerable research is under way to map the molecular steps involved in the above pathway, with the aim of developing therapeutic strategies to block the process of atherogenesis. However, a healthy diet, regular exercise and avoidance of tobacco would be a useful start to preventing this disease. Lifestyle improvements such as these are already having a beneficial effect in the West.

Infection by chlamydia and viruses such as herpes has been implicated as the initiating inflammatory stimulus, but an infective hypothesis remains unproven (Dongsheng et al., 1997), albeit interesting. The smooth muscle proliferation has been shown to be clonal (Benditt, 1988), but clonality *per se* is not a hallmark of neoplasia (see Chapter 24).

The main involvement of the anatomical pathologist with atherosclerosis is regrettably at autopsy. Because narrowing of coronary arteries is common, the pathologist must ensure that the extent of narrowing (if there is no complete occlusion by recent thrombosis) is sufficient to explain a sudden death. The pathologist may also be required to explain the mechanism of death following treatment of atheromatous arteries, for example by balloon angioplasty, vascular replacement or coronary artery bypass surgery.

ARTERIOLOSCLEROSIS

Arteriolosclerosis is a hyaline (glassy eosinophilic) thickening of the walls of arterioles that is age related but more severe and generalised in hypertensive subjects. Hypertension may be caused by a variety of hormone-secreting tumours, chronic renal diseases and vascular disorders including renal artery stenosis and polyarteritis nodosa. However, the essential cause is unknown in the vast majority of cases, although it is almost certainly polygenic (due to the interaction of several genes and environmental influences). The main complication of hypertension is accelerated atherogenesis leading to the outcomes described above. The major clinical sequelae are hemorrhagic stroke, aortic aneurysm and hypertensive and ischaemic heart disease.

Arteriolosclerosis is also seen in diabetics. The change is particularly evident in the arterioles of the kidneys, and leads to progressive ischaemic damage and symmetrical atrophy (shrinkage) of the kidneys (see Chapter 33).

VASCULITIS

Inflammatory injury of vessels (excluding atherosclerosis) that may be accompanied by necrosis of the vessel wall has many causes and clinical associations. The effects may be very widespread, and may produce a bewildering range of clinical signs and symptoms. The skin is often involved, and vessel wall necrosis will produce hemorrhagic spots (purpura). Other sites of damage include kidney, joints, gut and brain. Vasculitis may range from mild and self-limiting to severe and life-threatening.

Different types of vasculitis show a predilection for vessels of a particular type or size. It may be caused by the direct toxic effects of a variety of infective organisms (e.g. bacteria such as *Neisseria meningitidis*, and viruses such as herpes), by the deposition of immune complexes within the vessel wall (antigen—derived from hepatitis B for example— complexed with antibody), by direct antibody damage, or in association with antineutrophil cytoplasmic antibodies (ANCA). Each of the last three factors or processes affect small arteries, arterioles, capillaries or venules. The histopathological changes in small vessel vasculitis may be subtle, but include the presence of neutrophils and fibrin in the vessel wall and lumen, sometimes associated with neutrophil nuclear fragmentation within and outside the wall (leukocytoclasis).

The causes of giant cell (temporal) arteritis and classical polyarteritis nodosa, which affect large to medium-sized arteries are still unknown. Two rare causes of large vessel arteritis are Takayasu's disease (affecting the aorta and its branches in young women) and Kawasaki's disease (affecting medium-sized arteries including the coronary arteries in young children). Syphilitic arteritis involving the ascending aorta is now uncommon. In syphilis, chronic inflammation is focused on the vasa vasorum, the small vessels that enter through the adventitia to supply the outer part of the vessel. This leads to progressive weakening, aneurysmal dilatation and ultimately rupture of the aorta.

REFERENCES

Benditt, E.P. (1988) Origins of human atherosclerotic plaques: The role of altered gene expression. *Arch Pathol Lab Med,* **112**, 997–1001.

Campbell, J.H. & Campbell, G.R. (1994) The role of smooth muscle cells in atherosclerosis. *Current Opinion in Lipidology,* **5**, 323–330.

Dongsheng, Y., Nichols, T.C., Dehmer, G.J., Tate, D.A., Wehbie, R.S. & Quinlivan E.B. (1997) Absence of human herpes virus and genomes in coronary atherosclerosis in immunocompetent patients. *Am J Cardiol,* **79**, 1245–1247.

Moolenaar, W. & Lamers, C.B.H.W. (1996) Cholesterol crystal embolisation to the alimentary tract. *Gut,* **38**, 196–200.

Ross, R. & Fuster, V. (1996) In *Atherosclerosis and Coronary Artery Disease,* edited by V. Fuster, R. Ross & E.J. Topol, pp. 441–460. Philadelphia: Lippincott-Raven.

Stary, H.C. (1996) In *Atherosclerosis and Coronary Artery Disease,* edited by V. Fuster, R. Ross & E.J. Topol, pp. 463–465. Philadelphia: Lippincott-Raven.

Woolf, N. (1990) Pathology of atherosclerosis. *Br Med Bull,* **46**, 960–985.

— PART IV —

NEOPLASIA

20

THE NATURE AND CAUSE OF CANCER: HISTORICAL OVERVIEW

It is fear that I am most afraid of

Michel Montaigne

Why are there so many ideas about the origin and nature of cancer?

HUMORAL THEORIES

The word cancer originates from the writings of Hippocrates (c.450–370BC), who observed distended vessels radiating from a central lump in the breast like the legs of a crab (Cantor, 1993). *Cancer* in Latin or *Karkinoma* in Greek means crab. The earliest views on the nature of cancer relate to the 'humoral' theory of health and disease, which was developed in the world of ancient Greece and refined in the Roman period by the philosopher/physician Galen. This theory was dominant in Western medicine until the nineteenth century, and was also promulgated by the Arabs during the first millennium, with traces surviving in the Islamic world today. The humoral theory was holistic and has many similarities with Indian and Eastern medical traditions (Nutton, 1993). The word humour stems from a Greek word 'cumor' describing any form of fluid. To be in good humour originally related to the idea that a favourable balance of the four humours—black bile, yellow bile, blood and phlegm—was the basis of a pleasant mood. Disease was believed to be caused by the contamination of blood with other humours, particularly black bile. One could encourage healing by removing the contaminated blood, hence the widespread practice of blood letting or applying leeches to the skin.

Galen believed that cancer was the result of an excess of black bile, the same humour responsible for the state of melancholy (this word literally means black bile). The nature of blood, yellow bile and phlegm is now widely understood, but black bile is a much more mysterious substance. According to a number of ancient Greek authorities it is normally invisible, but 'bubbles and hisses when it touches the ground, destroying anything in its path' (Nutton, 1993). Conceivably it could have related to the altered blood that is vomited or passed rectally following internal haemorrhage. It could also have related to malignant melanomas since, although very rare, these cutaneous cancers would have been visible to Greek physicians. Galen advanced the view that an excess of black bile in the body might spill over into a local region to become a hard mass that either was a cancer from the outset or might develop later into a cancer.

CHEMICAL THEORIES

In the sixteenth and seventeenth centuries, chemical ideas were being applied to the practice of medicine (iatrochemistry). Paracelsus (1493–1541), the alchemist, physician and mystic, held views that were ahead of his time and introduced new remedies including opium, iron, laudanum, sulphur compounds, mercury and arsenic (all used in the following centuries and some to this day). Despite his background in occultism, Paracelsus rejected views of mental disease as a manifestation of demonic possession, and was probably the first to attack the humoral view of disease as nonsensical, emphasising his views by burning the works of Galen. Instead he contested that diseases including cancer were caused by toxic chemical agents such as 'noxious acids and ferments'.

Other alternatives to the humoral view were put forward from time to time. Following the discovery of the lymphatic system by the anatomist Gaspare Aselli (1581–1625), the lymphatic fluids and lymph nodes came to be associated with the development of cancer. Georg Stahl (1660–1734), an influential German chemist, concluded that black bile was a composite substance that included lymph mixed with small amounts of blood. Trapped in lymph nodes this resulted in an inflammatory ferment culminating in the development of cancer. This idea has not entirely disappeared in the twentieth century, with alternative practices envisaging the accumulation of 'toxins' within the lymphatic system that could either discharge harmlessly as inflammation or continue to solidify as a cancer. The sixteenth- and seventeenth-century idea of fermentation was linked to the proliferative ferments that occurred in bread and alcoholic beverages, and the obvious analogy with the growth of cancer. The Dutch physician Hermann Boerhaave (1668–1738) believed that blockage in the circulation of the blood was the key factor, this leading to inflammation and in turn to cancer (Cantor, 1993).

CELL THEORIES

The demise of the humoral and chemical theories came in the eighteenth and nineteenth centuries when the structure of the body was conceived as a set of different tissues. M. F. X. Bichat (1771–1802) advanced the view that different parts of the body containing the same type of tissue would develop similar disease processes and that cancer was fundamentally a disease of body tissues. This was a major step forward from the fluid–based view of disease, but more important still was the recognition of the cell as the unit of life (Bracegirdle, 1993).

Theodor Schwann (1810–1882) established the universal cell theory in 1839: the cell unit comprised a nucleus and surrounding cell sap enclosed by a wall. The cell sap was found to be contractile and glutinous, and was described as protoplasm (now known as cytoplasm) by Jan Purkinje (1787–1869). It was originally held that cells formed like crystals but in a biological medium called 'cytoblastema'. Microscopic techniques aided the recognition of replication of cells by division into two identical 'daughter' cells a number of years later. Walther Flemming (1843–1905) recognised the separation of chromosomes during cell division, introducing the term 'mitosis' to describe this process. Rudolf Virchow (1821–1902) was the first to appreciate that cancer was a disease of cells that grew through the process of cell division, but believed that cancers arose from 'embryonic' or primitive cells scattered throughout the connective tissue of the body. It was Wilhelm Waldeyer (1837–1921) who argued for the origin of cancers from the tissues with which they were associated, cancers of skin arising from the epithelium of the skin itself and cancers of the epithelium lining hollow organs arising from the same.

AETIOLOGY OF CANCER

Modern cancer research has focused on the cause and treatment of cancer, considerably extending our understanding of the nature of cancer. Theories on the cause of cancer have ranged from external agents in the form of infectious organisms, environmental chemicals and physical factors (notably radiation), to constitutional factors such as genetic mutations. It is now believed to be a combination of environmental and constitutional factors, though the abnormal behaviour of the malignant cell is explained by alteration or mutation of genetic material. (This is addressed further in Chapter 23.) Modern technology has also confirmed that a cancer is a clone of cells, meaning that all the malignant cells that form a cancer are descendants of a single cell.

The failure of modern medicine to curtail cancer has encouraged the popular belief that cancer is a 'whole body' disease caused by exposure to environmental factors such as toxins, psychological stress and the by-products of modern technology. Cancer is regarded by many as a recent disease, a product of the environment that the Western world has created in its blindness and ignorance. Contrasting with the common curse of cancer in the West is the perception of a virtual absence of the disease amongst animals living in the wild and according to the laws of nature. Whilst widely held, most of the preceding premises are fallacious. Human remains indicate the existence of cancer since the dawn of civilisation. Breast cancer is well documented in the literature of the Graeco–Roman period.

We are seeing more cancer now because it is (in general terms) an age-related disease, and people are now more likely to live to an advanced age. Today, a British woman can expect to live to be over 80. In the 1750s the median age at death for a British woman was 35 years (Anderson, 1987). The diagnosis is no longer being concealed as it was in the past when the word 'cancer' was considered taboo and deliberately omitted from death certificates. A diagnosis of cancer, including earlier diagnosis, is being made more readily through improvements in and increasing use of cancer screening methods. It is unusual for anyone to 'die merely of old age' as they commonly did in the past. Many forms of cancer are more common in the Third World than in the West, however, despite the lower life expectancy of Third World inhabitants (Boyle, 1997). Particular examples are cancers caused by infectious agents (e.g. hepatitis B and C, Epstein-Barr virus, human immunodeficiency virus and *Helicobacter pylori*). This is in part due to the high prevalence of these organisms in the Third World. Animals in the wild have a very limited life expectancy. Pet owners are well aware that cancer may be the cause of death in pets who through the benefits of modern civilisation are the Methuselahs of the animal kingdom.

Cancer of the lung is the leading cause of cancer death worldwide, the major cause being smoking. Most people who smoke will not get cancer, but 90% of people who get lung cancer have a long history of smoking. The ratio of male to female smokers in North America, northwest Europe and Australasia has gradually changed in favour of females over time. The incidence of lung cancer in males inhabiting these regions has plateaued out; conversely, the incidence of lung cancer amongst females is increasing. Genetic factors play a part, probably through the lack of protective genes as much as through the presence of harmful genes. Individuals lacking protective genes will be particularly sensitive to the cancer-causing compounds in cigarette smoke. As passive smokers, they will contribute to the 10% of non-active smokers who develop lung cancer.

The second most frequent cause of cancer death worldwide is gastric cancer, though the incidence of this cancer in the West has been falling steadily in the last one hundred years and continues to fall. The causes of gastric cancer are less clear than those of lung cancer, but it is now well established that nearly all those with cancer of the stomach develop the disease within a background of chronic inflammation of the stomach lining. This inflammation is in most cases caused by a bacterium called *Helicobacter pylori*, identified by Marshall and Warren as recently as 1984. As in the case of smokers, only a small proportion of individuals with inflammation of the stomach will ultimately develop cancer. Additional factors such as dietary intake and genetic influences will add to the risk of developing cancer. Nevertheless, eradication of *Helicobacter pylori* infection would (like the cessation of smoking in the case of lung cancer) lead to a marked reduction in the incidence of stomach cancer (Forman, 1996).

The most common cancer of all is skin cancer, though it rarely kills. The exception is the relatively rare pigmented form called malignant melanoma, though even this can be cured if diagnosed early. The single most important cause is sunlight (ultraviolet radiation) which leads to DNA damage. Failure to repair damaged DNA may result in cancer causing mutations. As with most cancers, genetic factors also play a part. Individuals with dark skins produce more melanin which shields the cells of the skin from the damaging effects of sunlight. People with pale skin lack functioning genes responsible for the production of melanin.

Human papillomavirus (HPV) is an additional cause of squamous cell carcinoma, notably of the cervix. HPV-16 and HPV-18 mediate their oncogenic effect through oncoproteins called E6 and E7. The latter inactivate the tumour suppressor genes *p53* and *Rb* respectively. Some individuals have a variant of the *p53* gene which is susceptible to degradation by E6, consequently these individuals are at much greater risk of cervical cancer (Storey et al., 1998). This is a example of an interaction between environmental and genetic factors leading to increased cancer susceptibility.

The preceding examples indicate very clearly that the causes of some of the most common and most dangerous forms of cancer (melanoma, lung and gastric cancer) are linked to physical agents such as sunlight, chemical compounds (such as those found in cigarette smoke) or infective agents. In each of these cancers genetic factors play a part also. Other types of cancer have a similar story, whereas breast and prostate cancers still lack an external cause.

The principal carcinogenic agents are not the product of the Industrial Revolution, with the notable exception of ionising radiation. Once the danger of radiation was understood, its effects were controlled or restricted to specific localities either through accidents or deliberate aggression. Background ionising radiation (partly cosmic and partly stemming from the earth, e.g. radon gas) can never be eliminated and will contribute to spontaneous mutation and therefore to cancer risk. A minority of cancers are related to industrial exposure, for example mesothelioma caused by asbestos, and bladder cancer in beta-naphthylamine exposed workers in the aniline dye and rubber industries. Nevertheless, the majority of carcinogens either existed before the evolution of humankind (e.g. sunlight, background radiation and microbes), or relate to social habits developed over hundreds if not thousands of years.

There is very little room for some of the increasingly popular notions regarding cancer and its causes, the chief of these being 'stress'. The idea that stress causes cancer is little more than a superstitious fear, which throughout history has itself been one of the most stressful factors of life along with famine, temperature extremes, plagues and violence. Indeed, modern civilisation is remarkable for the comparative lack of external stresses of this type.

The idea of stress causing disease was introduced by the Canadian physician Hans Selye (1907–1982) (Porter, 1993). Selye envisaged the slow build-up of disturbed functions leading ultimately to heart attacks, ulcers, raised blood pressure and any other complaint of unknown aetiology, including cancer. Many of the causes of these ailments are still unknown, but we now know that chronic peptic ulceration, correlated with stress in the past, is the result of infection of the stomach by the bacterium *Helicobacter pylori*.

Various invisible stresses have also been invoked to explain cancer, for example electromagnetic and 'other' radiation from power lines, wrist watches, dental amalgam, magnets, cell phones and so on. These are believed to disturb the natural harmonies and rhythms of the body. Such beliefs are popular not because they are new and trendy but because they relate to basic or instinctive human behaviour. The attitude of the French peasant of the eighteenth century was characterised by a deep-rooted mistrust of change. When an area of peasant France was visited by surveyors intent on producing a map of the region, the surveyors were stoned by the local peasants who decided that they were a group of sorcerers whose actions would lead to hailstorms that would damage their crops (Anderson, 1987). Any novelty, whether this be new crops such as maize, or inoculation against smallpox, was greeted with hostile resistance by the peasantry (forming the bulk of the population) of eighteenth-century Europe. The history of humankind is filled with popular belief regarding the evil of novelty. This is just as true today with the examples of power lines and cellular phones as it was in the past. As fast as one such belief is demonstrated as being nonsensical it is replaced by another and so on, with the underlying instinctive mistrust of novelty remaining the same.

The history of our understanding of cancer has been one of a peculiar blend of accurate and distorted observation, logical reasoning and imaginative theories. The last, whilst incorrect in the main, have resurfaced repeatedly within both mainstream medical history and popular mythology. The old idea of an excess of black bile causing both cancer and melancholia revisits us in the present with the view of stress, depression or guilt as the cause of cancer. We certainly do not know all there is to know about cancer, but medical science, as shown in the following chapters, possesses the tools and the understanding to explain all that can be known about the disease, even if this process takes another century to reach completion.

REFERENCES

Anderson, M.S. (1987) The structure of society. In *Europe in the Eighteenth Century 1713–1783* (3rd edn), pp. 25–71. London and New York: Longman.

Boyle, P. (1997) Global burden of cancer. *Lancet,* **349**(suppl II), 23–26.

Bracegirdle, B. (1993) The microscopical tradition. In *Companion Encyclopedia of the History of Medicine*, volume 1, edited by W.F. Bynum & R. Porter, pp. 102–119. London and New York: Routledge.

Cantor, D. (1993) Cancer. In *Companion Encyclopedia of the History of Medicine*, volume 1, edited by W.F. Bynum & R. Porter, pp. 537–561. London and New York: Routledge.

Forman, D. (1996) Helicobacter pylori and gastric cancer. *Scand J Gastroenterol* (Suppl), **220**, 23–26.

Marshall, B.J. & Warren, J.R. (1984) Unidentified curved bacilli in the stomach of patients with gastritis and peptic ulceration. *Lancet,* **1**, 1311–1315.

Nutton, V. (1993) Humoralism. In *Companion Encyclopedia of the History of Medicine*, volume 1, edited by W.F. Bynum & R. Porter, pp. 281–291. London and New York: Routledge.

Porter, R. (1993) Diseases of civilization. In *Companion Encyclopedia of the History of Medicine*, volume 1, edited by W.F. Bynum & R. Porter, pp. 585–600. London and New York: Routledge.

Storey, A., Thomas, M., Kalita, A., Harwood, C., Gardiol, D., Mantovani, F., Breuer, J., Leigh, I.M., Matlashewski, G. & Banks, L. (1998) Role of a *p53* polymorphism in the development of human papilloma-virus-associated cancer. *Nature*, **393**, 229–234.

21

VISUAL HALLMARKS OF CANCER

The eye is the lord of the senses

Leonardo da Vinci

Which visual features are common to most forms of cancer?

TISSUE DIAGNOSIS: THE GOLD STANDARD

The diagnosis of cancer may be suspected on the basis of a patient's symptoms and the findings on clinical examination. Imaging modalities such as computerised axial tomography (CAT), ultrasound scanning, magnetic resonance imaging (MRI) and barium studies may provide more reliable guides to diagnosis. A tissue diagnosis, however, is not only the gold standard, but includes information on the type of cancer and its likely behaviour. Although there are many types of cancer, all are characterised by the properties of uncontrolled growth, invasion and destruction of local tissues, as well as (with the exception of basal cell carcinoma of skin and cancers of the central nervous system) the ability to spread to distant sites (metastasis). The classification of cancer into types and grades will be described in Chapter 22 and the mechanisms of spread in Chapter 24. In this chapter we will consider the generic features of cancer at macroscopic and microscopic levels.

MACROSCOPIC APPEARANCES OF CANCER

Many cancers originate within epithelial surfaces, such as the epidermis of the skin or the mucosal lining of hollow organs such as the gut. Others arise from the epithelium of the fine ducts or glands found within 'solid' organs such as the prostate, breast or pancreas. The way we 'see' cancer is determined by its origin within a flat surface versus solid tissue. A cancer originating within surface epithelium can be viewed from above, whereas a cancer growing in a solid organ can only be seen properly when it is removed and sectioned.

Since cancer originates from a single cell and shows progressive growth, it will eventually develop into a local mass or lump. The term 'tumour' means a localised swelling, but has come through popular usage to imply a cancer. A clinically palpable lump could be an inflammatory lesion such as an abscess, a cyst, a developmental malformation or hamartoma, a hernia, a benign neoplasm or a malignant neoplasm (cancer). The term 'neoplasm' means a new growth with the implication that growth is autonomous and continues after the initiating event has been removed (Willis, 1952). The distinction between benign and malignant neoplasms is considered in more detail in the following chapter.

Appearances of malignant neoplasms of skin

In considering the macroscopic appearances of cancer, it is convenient to begin with the skin. The skin is the most common site for malignancy. However, because skin cancers are relatively innocuous (with the exception of malignant melanoma), cancer registries do not record their incidence. Skin cancers can be observed at a relatively early stage in their evolution. Non-malignant cutaneous lumps are also common and reveal useful distinguishing features from cancer.

In general terms, cancers arising from an epithelial surface are raised, flat or depressed. Excessive local growth that is associated with little local invasion must result in a mass that is raised above the level of the epithelium. Growth of this type is described as exophytic (growth upwards or outwards), and the resulting lesion may be referred to as polypoid or simply a polyp (particularly when a head is formed with a distinct stalk). One of the most common forms of skin cancer is the squamous cell carcinoma. This is typically an exophytic growth with a broad or sessile base. The surface is warty with irregular finger-like projections. Its size and a history of progressive growth will be indicators of malignancy. Basal cell carcinomas, also very common, may form a smooth, slightly raised and firm nodule. The centre may become depressed leaving a rounded, pearly edge. Some basal cell carcinomas remain flat and indistinct apart from causing thickening of the underlying tissues. These less nodular basal cell carcinomas tend to be multifocal and/or show diffuse infiltration of the dermis. Obvious ulceration (loss of epithelium) is relatively unusual in skin cancers, even in the case of aggressive malignant melanomas. This is because patients are generally treated when the cancer is at an early stage. Left untreated, however, a proportion of skin cancers will ulcerate. Some basal cell carcinomas will invade and destroy underlying tissues in such an aggressive manner that they have been called rodent ulcers (the unfortunate patient may look like the victim of a hungry rodent). Malignant melanoma is recognised by its changing appearance, with regard to size, colour (increase or decrease in pigmentation) and bleeding. It may be nodular or flat, the former being the more aggressive.

Should a skin cancer be left untreated and ulcerate, there will be bleeding or oozing of serum that forms a crust. With increasing size and excavation, the ulcer will not scab over like a skin wound, but the covering of granulation tissue will ooze or bleed and there may be infection with micro-organisms. An advanced skin cancer will produce extensive and distressing local destruction, and uncontrolled infection will result in offensive putrefaction of the underlying soft tissues. Surgery is not only aimed at curing cancer, but also at removing its visible manifestations which can be nothing short of horrific.

Benign cutaneous neoplasms and cysts

The 'innocent' skin lesions are too numerous to list in detail. In general they are small and show little or no discernible change over time and no evidence of bleeding (unless there has been obvious trauma). The most common benign skin 'tumours' are actinic (solar) keratoses, basal cell papillomas (seborrhoeic warts), dermatofibromas, pigmented nevi and sebaceous cysts. A cyst is a collection of fluid or semisolid material that is enclosed in a sac with an epithelial lining. Cysts are round and smooth but may feel extremely hard because of their accumulated contents. The scalp is a common site for sebaceous cysts. Cysts in superficial organs or tissues may be palpated through the skin, for example of testis and associated structures, thyroid or breast. Cysts may also occur in every internal organ. Neoplasms may include cystic areas, for example benign and malignant tumours of the ovary.

Malignant neoplasms in internal hollow organs

Cancers that occur in the epithelial lining of internal hollow organs such as the stomach or colon may not be noticed by the patient until they obstruct the organ (see Chapter 32) or ulcerate and bleed. By this time they will have reached a relatively large size, i.e. 3–15 cm in diameter. An obstruction of the large intestine is often due to cancer. Patients present with lower abdominal colicky pain and require immediate surgery. A cancer of the bronchus may ulcerate and bleed resulting in haemoptysis, or cause obstruction that leads to infection (pneumonia) presenting with general malaise, cough with purulent sputum and fever. Unlike cancer of skin, malignancy in an internal organ does not so much present as a lesion or mass which can be seen or felt, but rather with symptoms secondary to its complications.

As in the skin, cancers arising within the epithelial lining of a hollow organ may be protuberant, flat or ulcerating. They may also cause a narrowing or stricturing of the organ as a result of diffuse circumferential growth. Ulceration is present to some degree in all such cancers, regardless of whether they are polypoid, flat or stricturing. Ulcerating cancers have a rolled, raised, everted edge.

Malignant neoplasms in internal solid organs

Cancers arising in a small tube, duct or gland within a solid organ will form a lump or mass. Regardless of whether a cancer is in the form of an ulcer or a roughly spherical mass, it is often of a firm to hard consistency. This hardness is not caused by the cancer cells but by non-malignant tissue that is intermingled with the cancer cells. The non-malignant components consist of connective tissue known as stroma (derived from the Greek word meaning a mattress or sofa). One function of the connective tissue stroma is to channel blood vessels to the growing cancer cells. Cancer cells actually stimulate the proliferation of connective tissue and accompanying blood vessels by secreting growth factors, such as vascular endothelial growth factor (VEGF). Ultimately the connective tissue may come to occupy more space within a cancer than the cancer cells themselves. Connective tissue cells include fibroblasts which secrete collagen. Tendons such as the Achilles tendon are extremely hard, due to the presence of collagen arranged in long, parallel bundles. The stroma within a cancer often contains abundant collagen. Such a cancer feels hard and is described as desmoplastic ('hard-moulded').

Cancers infiltrate adjacent tissues in two ways. The mass of malignant cells may simply keep on increasing in number so that the cancer pushes out evenly in all directions. Conversely, cells may become mobile and stream out in tongues giving the cancer a holly-leaf configuration. The accompanying connective tissue tethers the cancer to the surrounding structures that it encounters on its outward journey. An advanced cancer of breast, for example, will often feel like a hard and relatively tethered mass (when examined clinically).

When removed by a surgeon and sectioned with a knife or scalpel, cancers are often white, like a scar or tendon. This simply reflects the large amount of collagen-rich connective tissue. Tongues of firm white tissue may be seen extending into the surrounding normal tissues. The macroscopic and microscopic appearances of specific cancers are considered in more detail in Chapters 9 and 22.

MICROSCOPIC FEATURES OF CANCER

The diagnostic acid test for a cancer is microscopic examination. No single feature is absolutely diagnostic of cancer; the pathologist makes the diagnosis in the same way that an art expert recognises a painting by van Gogh. Nevertheless, just as one can analyse the subject matter, brush strokes, colours and paint thickness that contribute to a van Gogh painting, so can one single out the individual microscopic features of a cancer.

At the microscopic level the normal tissues of the body are not arranged in a haphazard form but according to a regular architectural plan. For example, the ducts in the breast will branch regularly like the veins on a leaf. From the terminal ducts radiate tiny ductules surrounded by a cushion of connective tissue. This forms a distinct unit called a lobule. Cancer cells invade but do not necessarily cause obvious death or destruction of the invaded tissues. However, by their invasion of normal tissues, cancer cells create distinct patterns quite unlike that of normal tissues. These abnormal growth patterns are visible on low power microscopic examination (too low to see individual cells). This architectural overview of a cancer provides important diagnostic information. Invasion is generally evident by the presence of malignant cells in an inappropriate location. Epithelial tissues sit on a delicate basement membrane. Epithelial cancers may therefore be diagnosed when cells breach the basement membrane and pass into the underlying connective tissue.

The collagen-rich connective tissue stroma that is intermingled with the malignant epithelium is sufficiently different from any normal tissue to be a useful guide to the presence of cancer (even though it is not malignant itself). By means of adhesion molecules and molecular messengers (see Chapter 16) the stroma plays a critical role in moulding the form of the cancer. Stroma and cancer form a very close partnership (Ronnov-Jessen et al., 1996). The development of a cancer beyond the pinhead size of 1 mm requires the induction of angiogenesis or neo-vascularisation. The stroma provides the cancer with its supporting microvasculature, but cancers often outgrow their own blood supply. This is why cancers growing within a surface epithelium become ulcerated and solid cancers become necrotic. Necrosis is not specific for cancer, but its presence provides another important diagnostic clue.

In fact, by the time one has examined a specimen of cancer by naked eye and low power microscopic examination, the diagnosis is usually certain. However, another important entity is still available for study: the malignant cell itself. A normal cell of the body performs a specialised function and this is mirrored by a recognisable light microscopic structure. The size, shape and staining pattern of a cancer cell is different from its normal counterpart. The nucleus is generally larger than normal and occupies a greater proportion of the cytoplasm. The chromatin opens up from its usual uniformly dense state (heterochromatin) to form coarse clumps and condensations beneath the nuclear membrane (hyperchromatism) with intervening finely dispersed euchromatin. The nuclei vary in size, shape and staining characteristics (pleomorphism) (Fig. 26). In malignant cells nucleoli are increased in size and number,

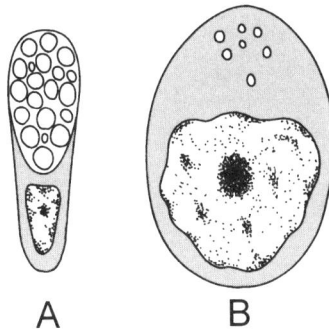

Figure 26 A: Normal columnar mucous cell. B: Adenocarcinoma cell containing a few secretory vesicles. The nucleus is enlarged, hyperchromatic and includes a large nucleolus.

reflecting the increased protein synthetic activity of the cell. One may be able to observe an unusually large number of cells in the process of division (mitosis). Appearances at the level of the individual cell are called cytological, as opposed to histological features at the tissue level. There is now an increasing tendency to achieve a cytological diagnosis of cancer by aspirating tiny fragments of tissue through a fine needle. While the information obtained will be less detailed and comprehensive than that achieved through a larger surgical biopsy, it will often be sufficient to guide further treatment.

This chapter has considered some of the clinical, naked eye and microscopic appearances of cancer, perhaps giving the impression that cancer is one disease that is able to attack different organs. In fact, although sharing common and recognisable characteristics, the cancers of different organs are very different diseases with differing causes and behaviours. Even within a single organ there may be different types of cancer (we have already referred to malignant melanoma, squamous cell carcinoma and basal cell carcinoma arising in the skin). The next chapter considers how the various types of cancer are recognised and classified.

REFERENCES

Ronnov-Jessen, L., Peterson, O.W. & Bissell, M.J. (1996) Cellular changes involved in conversion of normal to malignant breast: importance of the stromal reaction. *Physiol Rev*, **76**, 69–125.

Willis, R.A. (1952) *The Spread of Tumours in the Human Body*. London: Butterworth and Co.

22

THE MANY FACES OF NEOPLASIA

We must be absolutely certain of the nature of your primary tumour

Alexander Solzhenitsyn *(Cancer Ward)*

What is a neoplasm?

CANCER: A HETEROGENEOUS GROUP OF DISORDERS

Tuberculosis, whooping cough, gas gangrene and meningitis are all infectious diseases caused by a particular type of micro-organism: the bacterium. Yet we regard them as completely different diseases. Similarly, cancer encompasses a large group of disorders with different presentations, causes, treatments and outcomes. There are two aspects to the classification or coding of disease. First the name of the affected organ or region of the body is stated. Then the disease is named. Terms such as lung cancer, stomach cancer or skin cancer lack precision. Cancer must be typed in more detail using internationally agreed criteria and coding systems, promulgated by the World Health Organization (WHO) to ensure standardisation.

PRINCIPLES OF CLASSIFYING NEOPLASMS

Neoplasms, or new growths, represent a spectrum of lesions ranging from benign to malignant in their behaviour. It is traditional for textbooks to provide a definition of neoplasia along the lines of Willis (page 136), and then proceed to list the differences between benign and malignant neoplasms (Table 5). This tradition has generated problems and is now looking increasingly jaded. The term benign simply means that the lesion is not dangerous because it generally lacks any significant capacity for invading local tissues and, most importantly, does not spread to distant sites. A few may nevertheless kill by virtue of their origin in vital sites such as the brain.

It can be stated that in comparison with malignant neoplasms, benign neoplasms are more likely to be small, slow-growing, well circumscribed and similar in microscopic structure to the tissue of origin. Benign tumours are often stated to be encapsulated, but this applies only to

Table 5 Characteristics of benign versus malignant neoplasms

Benign	Malignant
Non-metastasising	Metastasising
Rarely lethal	Potentially lethal
Small size	Large size
Well circumscribed	Infiltrative margins
Sometimes encapsulated	Non-encapsulated
May be cystic	Usually solid
Well differentiated	Loss of differentiation
Few mitoses	Many mitoses
No necrosis	Necrosis

a small subset of those growing within solid organs or connective tissues. The capsule is usually little more than a thin layer of compressed connective tissue derived from the surrounding structures. The majority of benign neoplasms develop within epithelial surfaces and are not encapsulated.

The distinction between a benign and malignant neoplasm would seem to be of practical and fundamental importance. However, in the case of common neoplasms (the vast majority), the pathologist passes directly to the final diagnosis without troubling to identify all the features indicative of benign or malignant behaviour. The final diagnosis conveys prognostic significance because the behaviour of most types of neoplasm (benign or malignant) is well established. When the pathologist encounters a new or rare entity, however, it will be necessary to revisit the fundamental characteristics of benign versus malignant tumours. There are a number of neoplasms that, even today, cannot be categorised as being benign or malignant, but fall into a borderline category. It is usual to place some ovarian neoplasms and neoplasms derived from smooth muscle within this borderline group.

The main problem with the concept of benign neoplasia is the definition of neoplasia itself. No fewer than seven chapters of this book provide perspectives on neoplasia, including new insights relating to clonality and cancer genetics (see Chapters 23 and 24). Benign neoplasia does not encompass a single class of lesion. Some are precancerous, representing the early or pre-invasive stage of malignant neoplasms (e.g. adenoma to adenocarcinoma of the gastrointestinal tract or actinic keratosis to squamous cell carcinoma of the skin). Others, such as lipomas and angiomas, never become malignant. Then there are those lesions that have traditionally been regarded as non-neoplastic (perhaps described as hyperplastic, metaplastic, regenerative, cystic or hamartomatous), but, as shown by current research, are turning out to be clonal (derived from a single cell) and initiated by mutations implicating cancer genes. The modern reappraisal of proliferative lesions based upon the study of molecular mechanisms must nevertheless be tempered by knowledge of their clinical behaviour gathered over many years.

The classification of cancer is related to the concept of the body being formed of different types of tissue. The various tissues of the body have specific functions and specific structures. Similarly, the cells that form these tissues are of a particular size and shape, and will have some functions but not others. Mature cells are generated from precursor cells that lack specialised structure and function (stem cells). The development of an uncommitted stem cell into specialised daughter cells (perhaps two or more types of daughter cell) is described as differentiation (see Chapter 16). Although cancers show disordered structure and function, it is generally possible to observe differentiation into a particular type of tissue by the cancer cells. The type of cancer is therefore determined by the direction of differentiation taken by its constituent cells. Usually this direction is congruent with the tissue of origin. For example, a cancer arising in the epithelium of the skin (epidermis) looks somewhat like normal epidermis. However, the classification is based on the appearance taken by the cancer itself and not on the assumed tissue of origin. This approach is called a histogenetic classification (based on the tissues generated by the cancer).

HISTOGENETIC CLASSIFICATION OF NEOPLASMS

In order to apply a histogenetic classification to cancer, one needs to know about the structure and function of all the normal tissues of the body. It is beyond the scope of this book to give a detailed account of the normal body tissues, but an overview of the principles will suffice for the purposes of explaining cancer classification. Two major classes of tissue were mentioned in the previous chapter: epithelium and connective tissue. There are four types of epithelium: stratified squamous, columnar, cuboidal and transitional (Fig. 27).

Squamous cell neoplasms

The term 'stratified' means that the cells are piled up like the bricks of a wall. Those nearest the top become flattened like slates and are shed. Stratified squamous epithelium occurs in the skin, mouth, oesophagus, vagina and ectocervix. The most common type of cancer occur-

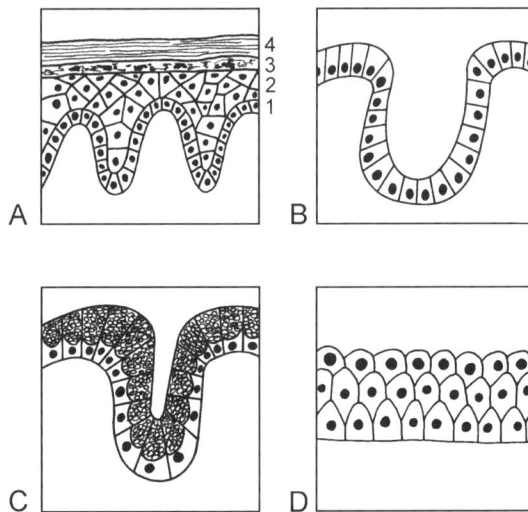

Figure 27 Types of epithelium. A: Stratified squamous epithelium (1 = basal cells, 2 = prickle cells, 3 = granular layer, 4 = keratinised or cornified layer). B: Cuboidal epithelium. C: Columnar epithelium. D: Transitional epithelium.

ring in all these sites is a squamous cell carcinoma. In the skin, the flattened cells accumulate a protein within their cytoplasm called keratin. The cells in all squamous epithelia are tightly held together by patches of adhesion molecules forming junctions called desmosomes. These specialised characteristics ensure the squamous epithelium is relatively tough and water-proof. Keratin production and desmosomes may be seen in squamous cell carcinomas of all sites, even those in which their normal counterpart does not produce abundant keratin (e.g. in sites such as the oesophagus and cervix).

Squamous cell carcinomas may also occur in areas where squamous epithelium is not found under normal circumstances. Lung cancers arising from the bronchial tree may be squamous, yet bronchi are lined by a specialised columnar type of epithelium or respiratory epithelium. The cells have whip-like cilia at their apex which are similar in structure to the tail of a sperm. These are only just visible under the microscope. Their wave-like coordinated motion wafts inhaled particles out of the lungs and up into the throat. The particles are trapped within mucus secreted by a second class of columnar cell called a goblet cell. In smokers and individuals with chronic lung disease this respiratory epithelium may be re-placed by a squamous epithelium, a process described as metaplasia (Greek for 'moulding a different form'). A diagnosis of squamous cell carcinoma of the lung may be suspected macroscopically because of the yellow colour of accumulated keratin. Squamous cell carcino-mas are graded histologically (well, moderate and poor) on the basis of differentiation towards keratin production.

Glandular neoplasms

Columnar epithelium lines the gastrointestinal tract (stomach, small intestine and large intes-tine) as well as the lung. The gut serves to absorb nutrients but also secretes mucus and digestive enzymes. Tissues that secrete are described as glandular and a simple gland is shaped like a microscopic flask or test tube and is lined by columnar or cuboidal epithelium. The secretions pass into the central space or lumen of the gland and then pour into the gut cavity. Carcinomas arising in such glandular tissues are called adenocarcinomas, and are recognised by the presence of gland-like structures which secrete mucus. Cystic spaces with mucoid contents may be apparent on gross inspection of the cut surface. Adenocarcinomas also arise from solid (as opposed to tube-like) organs that are essentially glandular in struc-ture. Examples are the prostate, pancreas, breast and endocrine glands. Adenocarcinomas are graded as well, moderately and poorly differentiated on the basis of gland formation (Fig. 28).

Transitional cell neoplasms

Transitional epithelium lines the renal pelvis, ureter, urinary bladder and urethra. This epithe-lium is stratified like squamous epithelium, but there are fewer layers of cells and the cells are plumper. Cancers arising in the urinary tract are usually transitional cell carcinomas. They are typically papillary growths with delicate seaweed-like fronds.

All cancers (malignant neoplasms) arising from epithelial surfaces or glands are carcino-mas of one type or another. Benign neoplasms also occur in these sites. Those arising in squamous or transitional epithelium are often called papillomas whereas adenomas occur in glandular tissues such as those of the gut lining, or solid organs such as the liver or the various endocrine glands (Table 6).

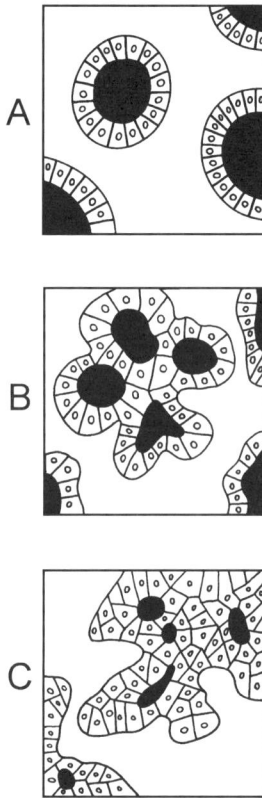

Figure 28 Adenocarcinoma. A: Well differentiated with simple tubules. B: Moderately differentiated with irregular tubules. C: Poorly differentiated with loss of tubular architecture.

Table 6 Classification of neoplasms of epithelial origin

Epithelium of origin	Benign	Malignant
Squamous	Papilloma	Squamous cell carcinoma
Transitional	Papilloma	Transitional cell carcinoma
Glandular	Adenoma	Adenocarcinoma

Note: Papilloma is derived from the term papilla and describes a small nipple-like lesion that is elevated or projects above the epithelial surface. Lesions with finger or leaf-like processes composed of epithelium overlying a fibrovascular core are described as papillary (e.g. papillary transitional cell carcinoma of urinary bladder) or as villous (e.g. villous adenoma of gut).

NEOPLASMS OF MESENCHYME

The term sarcoma refers to a cancer arising from mesenchymal tissue. The prototypic mesen-chymal derivative is connective tissue, the supporting layer that underlies epithelia and surrounds ducts. This kind of connective tissue (or stroma) has a loose texture because the cells (fibroblasts) are widely scattered in a mucoid matrix that includes collagen fibres that are secreted by the fibroblasts. Cancers arising in such tissue may be termed fibrosarcomas and are characterised by the presence of collagen fibres. However, the term connective tissue can be broadened to encompass more specialised types of tissue of mesenchymal origin, includ-ing muscle, fat and bone. It is very unusual for adult skeletal muscle to become malignant, but the smooth muscle found in the gut, walls of blood vessels or uterus (over which we have no voluntary control) may give rise to cancers. Cancers of smooth muscle, fat and bone are called leiomyosarcomas, liposarcomas and osteosarcomas respectively. The benign equiva-lents are leiomyomas, lipomas and osteomas (Table 7). Many sarcomas are white and soft on sectioning, rather like the flesh of fish.

Some benign connective tissue tumours (the term benign implying that they have no ability to spread to distant sites) show diffuse infiltration of surrounding tissues and very wide surgical excision is required to prevent local recurrence of the growth. Examples are the fibromatoses which, in view of their unique behaviour and appearance, have traditionally been considered as non-neoplastic (though have now been shown to demonstrate clonal genetic changes). This emphasises the practical importance of correct histological typing, and of the translation of this information into appropriate therapeutic action. The problems associated with distinguishing benign and malignant neoplasms have already been discussed. We can add the fact that the criteria for distinguishing benign and malignant neoplasms differ for the various types of neoplasm.

Haematological neoplasms

The third major category of cancer encompasses the haematological malignancies: leukaemia and lymphoma. Leukemia arises from the bone marrow, which is responsible for generating

Table 7 Classification of non-epithelial and special neoplasms

Tissue of origin	Benign	Malignant
Fibrous (connective tissue)	Fibroma	Fibrosarcoma
Fat	Lipoma	Liposarcoma
Smooth muscle	Leiomyoma	Leiomyosarcoma
Striated muscle	Rhabdomyoma	Rhabdomyosarcoma
Cartilage	Chondroma	Chondrosarcoma
Bone	Osteoma	Osteosarcoma
Blood vessels	Haemangioma	Haemangiosarcoma
Lymphoid	–	Lymphoma
Germ cell	Benign teratoma	Malignant teratoma
	–	Seminoma
Neuroectoderm	Nevus	Melanoma

red blood cells and most of the white blood cells found in the circulation. Lymphomas arise within lymph nodes, the spleen or the more diffuse masses of extranodal mucosa associated lymphoid tissue such as the tonsils. Hodgkin's disease is a particular type of lymphoma. All lymphomas are malignant; benign tumours of lymphoid tissue are not recognised, though some lymphomas are very slow-growing and, particularly in the elderly, pose little or no threat to health. Lymphomas are typically white, soft and homogeneous on sectioning.

OTHER TYPES OF NEOPLASM

The majority of cancers may be ascribed to one of the three cancer types: carcinoma, sarcoma and lymphoma. This classification has an embryological basis. When an ovum is fertilised by a sperm, the result is a single cell or zygote (from the Greek word meaning joined together). The zygote carries the potential to form all the cells of the body. At first this totipotential cell divides to form two, then four, then eight cells and so on. At this early stage the ball of cells may be disaggregated and could in theory form a clone of two, four, eight or sixteen identical individuals. The embryo starts to form when groups of cells become committed to a particular line of tissue differentiation, of which there are three major types. Ectoderm forms the skin and nervous system, endoderm forms the epithelial lining of internal hollow organs (e.g. gut) and associated glandular organs (e.g. liver and pancreas), and mesoderm forms all the rest (muscle, bone, bone marrow, cartilage, lymphoid system and connective tissue). As a general rule carcinomas arise from ectoderm or endoderm, whereas sarcomas and lymphomas arise from mesoderm.

A few types of cancer have not been mentioned. Most of these, however, are logically grouped with the carcinomas. Malignant melanomas are related developmentally to a specialised ectoderm which supports the differentiation of the nervous system (neuroectoderm). Malignant tumours occurring in early childhood often show a microscopic resemblance to tissues found in the normal embryo. These tumours are called blastomas, the term 'blast' signifying an immature type of cell. Examples are hepatoblastoma of the liver, retinoblastoma of the eye, nephroblastoma of the kidney, medulloblastoma of the brain and neuroblastoma of the peripheral nervous system. Most adult nervous system tumours are derived not from nerve cells but from 'supporting' cells such as astrocytes and oligodendrocytes. Mesotheliomas are derived from the mesothelial lining of serous membranes such as the pleural sacs. Malignant mesotheliomas are mesodermal in origin but mimic adenocarcinoma microscopically.

There is a final category of tumour that is distinct. Neoplasms may arise from germ cells that give rise to ova or sperm. Germ cells lack the commitment of cells found in ectoderm, mesoderm or endoderm. When a germ cell becomes neoplastic there are two possible outcomes: there may be no differentiation at all so that the cancer consists exclusively of dividing germ cells (seminoma in testis or dysgerminoma in ovary), or the germ cells may differentiate into all three embryonic (or germ) tissues: ectoderm, mesoderm and endoderm. Differentiation may reach a very high level with the formation of skin, hair, teeth and brain tissue! Such a tumour is called a teratoma and may be benign or malignant. Germ cell cancers occur in the ovary and testis and sometimes in other parts of the body (the thymus, pineal region and, in neonates, the sacro-coccygeal region).

The histogenetic classification provides more than a mere categorisation of cancer. It groups cancers into types that differ in terms of their causation, presentation, treatment and outcome. For example, it could be said that lung cancer is caused by smoking. This is virtually always true for squamous cell carcinoma, but less so for adenocarcinoma of the lung which is caused by other factors also. There is a third category of lung cancer called oat cell carcinoma (see below), which tends to disseminate widely so that surgery is attempted in a minority of cases only. Most patients with oat cell carcinoma of the lung die within a year of diagnosis, whereas the other lung cancers may be cured by surgery. Thus, the term lung cancer or carcinoma is not a complete diagnosis. The range of cancers occurring within each organ or system is large and coverage goes beyond the scope of this book (Fletcher, 1996).

POORLY DIFFERENTIATED CANCER

It is fortuitous that most cancers do differentiate into a recognisable tissue type which is generally congruent with the tissue of origin. Unfortunately this is a rule which cancers are at liberty to break. In a series of cancers of one type (e.g. adenocarcinoma of the colon) some will be well-differentiated, closely resembling the tissue of origin. At the other extreme will be cancers that can only just be recognised for what they are (Fig. 28). Cancers that closely resemble the tissue of origin (well-differentiated) tend to be the least aggressive in their behaviour, whilst the opposite is true of poorly differentiated cancers. However, there are also cancers that are undifferentiated or so poorly differentiated that typing is not possible. For example, it may be difficult to decide whether a cancer is a carcinoma, a sarcoma or a lymphoma. This is a very practical problem because the treatment and outcome of a cancer is determined by its underlying type. But how do we manage cancer that is apparently undifferentiated?

It was thought that the invention of the electron microscope would overcome the problem of the undifferentiated cancer. Indeed it was originally believed that the thousandfold increased magnification of this instrument would render the light microscope completely obsolete (Bracegirdle, 1993). The specialised structure and function of a cell is revealed in fine detail by the electron microscope, allowing faint traces of differentiation to be discerned in seemingly undifferentiated cells at this high level of magnification. For example, at the electron microscope level, oat cell carcinoma of the lung is found to contain hormonal secretory granules. Nevertheless, there will always be a residue of cancers that is undifferentiated even when cells are magnified a millionfold.

More subtle than ultrastructural features visible at the electron microscopic level is the molecular signature of a cell's state of structure and function. To read the molecular signature one would require probes that are specific for certain molecules and a system for amplifying a signal that might be relatively weak in the case of an undifferentiated cell. This tool arrived in the form of immunohistochemistry, boosted by the development of monoclonal antibody technology (see Chapter 3). Using monoclonal antibodies generated against molecules that are unique to cells of a particular type it is now possible to assign over 99% of cancers to a correct histogenetic classification (Table 8). It should be stressed that immunohistochemistry is only necessary for the investigation of a minor subset of cancers. Routine H&E sections are perfectly adequate for the great majority of tumour diagnoses.

MIXED NEOPLASMS

Most neoplasms can be classified according to the principles outlined above into histogenetic (tissue-based) types, and (in the case of malignant neoplasms) graded according to the level of malignancy (see below). The fact that cancers can be classified like animals or plants indicates a degree of behavioural predictability in relation to a disease that is perceived as being anarchic. Nevertheless, there are always exceptions to rules. In relation to the type of tissue constituting a neoplasm, some benign and malignant tumours (other than germ cell tumours) may be composed of a combination of epithelial and connective tissue components. It should be stressed that the connective tissue in this situation is not merely reactive host response forming a supporting stroma, but appears to be neoplastic in its own right, an integral part of the growth. How can this be if a cancer is derived from ectoderm, mesoderm or endoderm, and conforms to the underlying laws of differentiation governing these germ tissues? There are several explanations. Firstly, the epithelial component may in fact be an innocent bystander in what is actually a connective tissue neoplasm. This applies to the most common form of benign breast neoplasm known (ambiguously) as a fibroadenoma. The connective tissue or fibrous component of this tumour is monoclonal, whereas the entrapped epithelial component is polyclonal (like normal ductal epithelium).

Secondly, neoplasms may be derived from cells that originate in ectoderm yet in themselves show evidence of hybrid or ambivalent differentiation. An example of this is the myoepithelial cell (found in the ducts of various glands), which is epithelial in origin yet contains cellular components (such as contractile smooth muscle filaments) that are characteristic of cells of mesodermal origin. Such cells give rise to the common benign tumour of salivary glands called (appropriately) a mixed tumour.

Finally, it should be recalled that whilst mesoderm is associated with the various connec-

Table 8 Monoclonal antibodies commonly used in the diagnosis of the major classes of malignant tumours

Tumour type	Monoclonal antibody specificity
Carcinoma	Cytokeratin, epithelial membrane antigen (EMA)
Adenocarcinoma	Carcinoembryonic antigen (CEA)
Lymphoma	Leucocyte common antigen (LCA) (CD45)
B cell	CD20, CD45RA, CDw75, light chains (κ), (λ)
T cell	CD3, CD43, CD45RO
Sarcoma	Vimentin
Muscle	Desmin
Vessels	CD31, factor VIII
Melanoma	S100, HMB45
Germ cell	
Seminoma	Placental alkaline phosphatase (PLAP)
Yolk sac	Alpha fetoprotein (αFP)
Choriocarcinoma	Human chorionic gonadotrophin (HCG)
Neuroendocrine	Chromogranin

tive tissues of the body, a number of glandular organs or tissues are derived from this germ layer, for example the kidneys, the endometrial lining of the uterus and the mesothelium of serous membranes. Therefore it is only to be expected that neoplastic mesoderm should be capable of bidirectional differentiation to form both epithelial and connective tissues. Carcinomas of ectodermal or endodermal origin may rarely contain sarcomatous-appearing (malignant connective tissue) elements and have been described as carcinosarcomas. However, the behaviour of these tumours generally fits with the underlying carcinoma and not with the sarcomatous component.

PRIMARY AND SECONDARY (METASTATIC) CANCER

A tumour of the skin which looks somewhat like normal skin is likely to have arisen in the skin. Conversely a tumour of the skin that looks like a cancer of the breast or kidney probably did not arise in the skin but spread from the breast or kidney. In other words, such a growth is not a primary cancer but a secondary deposit of cancer or a metastasis. It is important to know if a growth is primary or secondary because treatment will be very different. Radical surgery for a secondary deposit of cancer is generally, though not always, inappropriate, because such a deposit indicates that the cancer is no longer localised. Apart from histogenetic clues, metastatic deposits tend to be multiple and spherical. Histologically they are rarely associated with any inflammatory host reaction. Mechanisms of metastasis are considered in Chapter 24.

GRADING OF CANCER

Two major elements in the diagnosis of cancer have not been addressed. One of these, the extent of spread, is discussed in Chapter 24. The other is the 'grade' of malignancy. In grading a cancer one is explaining behaviour or predicted behaviour in terms of one or more biological variables. There are traditional as well as recently recognised variables that have come to the fore with the advent of monoclonal antibody and molecular technology. Most of the traditional variables arose out of the visual hallmarks and histogenetic typing of cancer. Put simply, if one of the microscopic characteristics of cancer is present to a very marked degree, then the cancer is likely to be more aggressive. For example, in Chapter 21 it was stated that mitotic activity is a diagnostic hallmark of some cancers. In such cancers, a high rate of cell division might be worse for the patient than a low rate of cell division. There are some cancers, therefore, in which the counting of mitotic figures yields useful prognostic information (such as malignant melanoma, breast cancer and sarcomas). In other cancers, the rate of cell division is completely uninformative (e.g. in most adenocarcinomas).

Invasion of normal tissues is an important characteristic of cancer. Cancers that infiltrate normal tissues in a wide and diffuse fashion are more aggressive than those which tend to push out with a broad front (Fig. 29). This is a second prognostically useful feature, particularly in carcinomas, but is not helpful for lymphoma or sarcoma. Third is an immune response in the form of lymphocytes occurring in large numbers in and around a cancer. This serves as a sign of a favourable prognosis in adenocarcinomas of breast and colon and malignant melanoma. Marked variation in the size, shape and staining characteristics of nuclei is a fourth feature and is used in grading of breast carcinoma and sarcomas. A fifth feature is the degree of cellular or tissue differentiation as discussed above.

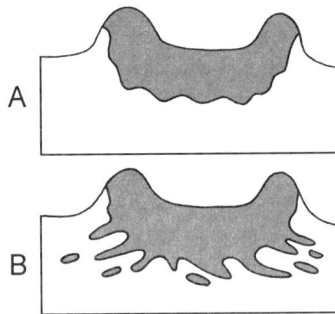

Figure 29 Sections through an ulcerated adenocarcinoma showing possible growth patterns. A: Pushing or relatively well circumscribed. B: Diffusely infiltrating.

For some cancers, two or more features are combined to give an overall score or biological grade. In breast cancer, the number of dividing cells in a defined area, the degree of glandular differentiation of the malignant cells and the variation in nuclear characteristics are combined into an overall index of cancer grade. Such prognostic indices based upon grading are not arbitrary, but depend on the demonstration that each variable provides unique or independent insight into outcome. The combination of two or more independent variables will often yield a prognosis that is extremely accurate. However, for an individual patient, prognosis is expressed as a survival probability rather than as an absolute certainty of outcome.

TUMOUR HETEROGENEITY

Heterogeneity may relate to the grade of a cancer as well as to the various types of tissue found in mixed tumours. Some parts of the tumour may be well-differentiated or low-grade, whereas subclones may have developed that are high-grade or poorly differentiated. Should the final grade be based on the 'worst' area (the most poorly differentiated), or the dominant area? To make such a decision one needs to follow the course of tumours of the same type that have been graded in both ways. Time will then tell which was the correct approach. This is much harder than it sounds, since it will be necessary to follow up many patients over several years before a clear pattern emerges. It has been assumed, however, that grading should generally be based upon the worst area. The fact that this has been generated in a less aggressive part of the same tumour should be immaterial if the worst part determines the overall clinical behaviour. Notable exceptions to this rule are cancers of prostate and testis.

NEW PROGNOSTIC MARKERS

Newer bio-markers relate either to altered genes or to the expressed products of genes within the nucleus, cytoplasm or cell membrane (Hermanek et al., 1995). Surprisingly, the 'big' science of the present has not eclipsed the old craft of the past. By the time we know the type, grade and extent of spread of a cancer, there is little room for additional prognostic information. In a sense this is not surprising if we perceive cancer as a form of behaviour resulting from genetic dysfunction. If one gene is mutated in one cancer but not in another, then the cancer without the mutation will make up for this by having a mutation in a different gene. Much of the modern approach to molecular diagnosis is demonstrating that there is more than one way to skin a cat. The markers that do provide useful information are those that relate to treatment decisions. For example, breast cancer cells that express oestrogen receptors will be stimulated by oestrogen and therefore suppressed by treatment with the anti-oestrogen drug tamoxifen. It has therefore become routine practice to look for oestrogen receptors in breast cancers by means of immunohistochemistry (see Chapter 3). It is likely that new molecular insights will lead more to treatment breakthroughs than to major changes in the practice of anatomical pathology, and that the application of the diagnostic gold standard provided by anatomical pathology will continue to underpin medical advances in the future.

REFERENCES

Bracegirdle, B. (1993) The microscopical tradition. In *Companion Encyclopedia of the History of Medicine*, volume 1, edited by W.F. Bynum & R. Porter, pp. 102–119. London and New York: Routledge.

Fletcher, C.D.M. (1995) (ed) *Diagnostic Histopathology of Tumors*, volume 1 and 2. Edinburgh: Churchill Livingstone.

Hermanek, P., Gospodarowicz, M.K., Henson, D.E., Hutter, R.V.P. & Sobin, L.H. (eds) (1995) *Prognostic Factors in Cancer*. Berlin: Springer.

Further reading

Rosai, J, & Sobin, L.H. (eds) (1991–1996) *Atlas of Tumor Pathology*, 3rd Series, Fascicles 1–18. Washington DC: Armed Forces Institute of Pathology.

World Health Organization. International Histological Classification of Tumours. 2nd series (1989–1998). Berlin, Heidelberg: Springer-Verlag.

23

CANCER: A GENETIC DISEASE

There is nothing hidden under the sun

Leonardo da Vinci

How do we know that cancer is a genetic disease?

GENETIC AND EPIGENETIC MECHANISMS

In the 1970s, opinion was divided as to whether cancer was fundamentally a genetic disease or arose through mechanisms independent of genetic alteration (epigenetic). The difference between genetic and epigenetic can be explained by analogy with a poor musical perform- ance. Likely explanations for a disagreeable sound would be errors by the musicians, snapped strings or poorly tuned instruments. These would all be 'epigenetic'. One would hardly expect that someone had managed to tamper with the musical score, replacing some notes with others— literally altering the code. The latter would be equivalent to a genetic alteration or mutation. In the 1980s, evidence that cancer was in fact a genetic disease began to accumu- late, implying the presence of changes within genes rather than in cellular mechanisms involved in translating and coordinating the encoded message. By the 1990s, three major classes of cancer gene had been identified: oncogenes, tumour suppressor genes and DNA repair genes. These insights were of paramount importance and required the convergence of four major disciplines: virology, genetics, molecular biology and anatomical pathology. Central to this was the participation of members of cancer families in which there was obvious transmis- sion of cancer risk from generation to generation.

ONCOGENES

In the first half of this century a number of studies had shown that particular viruses could cause cancer in selected animals. These were called oncogenic (cancer causing) viruses. In many instances, the genetic material contained within oncogenic viruses was RNA rather than DNA (see Chapter 27 for a brief account of DNA). To produce cancers in animals or humans these viruses would need to convert their RNA genes into DNA genes. The latter would then be integrated, and thereby hidden, within the DNA of the cell infected with the virus (Sambrook et al., 1968). The virus particle itself would disappear in this hit-and-run process. This description of viral parasitism is not only sinister, but does not fit with the traditional view that envisages DNA being transcribed into RNA, and not the other way round. However, Baltimore (1970) and Temin and Mizutani (1970) showed that RNA containing oncogenic viruses produced an enzyme reverse transciptase (hence retroviruses) that could indeed convert RNA into DNA.

It is now well accepted that certain viruses are responsible for causing particular human cancers. These include: human immmunodeficiency virus (HIV) and human T-cell lymphotropic virus-1 (both retroviruses) as causes of lymphoma; Epstein-Barr virus causing Burkitt lymphoma and nasopharyngeal carcinoma; hepatitis viruses B and C causing hepatocellular carcinoma; human papillomavirus causing cervical cancer and other squamous cell carcinomas; and herpes virus 8 causing Kaposi's sarcoma.

The relation between viral genes and cancer is clearly of importance, but research in this area drew attention to a still more important issue. Genes that were similar if not identical to the cancer genes of viruses were shown not to be exclusive to viruses but to reside in the cells of all species, including humans! The idea that we each carry genes that can cause cancer seems very strange until we realise that this is not the normal function of such genes. To cause cancer these genes need to be altered or mutated. The non-mutated genes are called proto-oncogenes, which are a large family responsible for the regulation of cell division (page 101). Oncogenes are mutated proto-oncogenes that may cause excessive cell division, one of the characteristics of a cancer cell. In summary, oncogenes can either be inserted into our cells by certain viruses, viral oncogenes (v-*onc*), or more commonly are the mutated forms of proto-oncogenes normally present within cells, cellular oncogenes (c-*onc*).

The oncogene theory vindicated the early suggestion made by Theodor Boveri (1862–1915) that cancer was caused by chromosomal alterations within the cells of the body (Cantor, 1993), and cancer can today be viewed as a disorder lying at the level of the gene, literally a genetic disease. The term genetic is not equivalent to the term hereditary. Although we inherit our genes from our parents and these genes sometimes contain disease-causing mutations, most of the genetic mutations that cause cancer are acquired in adult life. They are termed somatic mutations, the term somatic referring to any cell of the body with the exception of germ cells that give rise to sperm and ova.

Although cancer could in theory be caused by mutations in one or more of the numerous proto-oncogenes, it soon became clear that this class of genes was by no means the only one implicated in the causation of cancer. The discovery of two additional and very important classes of cancer gene was a by-product of the study of very rare hereditary forms of cancer.

INHERITED CANCER AND TUMOUR SUPPRESSOR GENES

The field of inherited disease is associated with a considerable number of difficulties. Inherited diseases are rare, usually untreatable, often amount to a terrible physical and psychological burden for affected individuals and their families and pose multiple ethical and cultural problems. The medical profession has generally preferred to avoid the issue of inherited cancer, mainly by denying its existence until recent times. It is true that cancer cells themselves are not transmitted from parent to child. Rather it is the transmission of particular mutated genes that serves to increase the probability that cancer will develop in individuals carrying the mutated gene. Even this concept has been met with resistance, clusters of the same cancer within a family being rationalised as coincidence or exposure to a similar environment. Where the inheritance of specific cancers has been acknowledged, it has often been as a grudging acceptance of the exception that proves the rule.

An example of a rare hereditary cancer is retinoblastoma, a cancer arising in children that develops in the retina. Knudson (1971) suggested that a particular type of genetic mechanism could explain the inheritance of retinoblastoma. Rather than growth being stimulated by a mutation in a single gene (e.g. an oncogene whose effects dominate over the remaining normal gene), he suggested that there could be inactivation or loss of both copies (maternal and paternal) of the same gene. An inactive copy of the causative gene could thereby be passed by one parent to every cell of the child. This would not matter until one of the cells within the retina lost its normal (or wild type) gene, leaving the cell with no functioning genes. An effect that requires loss of both genes is called recessive. It is recessive at the level of the affected cell. However the condition of retinoblastoma is dominant at the level of the family, since transmission of only one mutated gene is sufficient for the inevitable development of cancer in a child who carries the gene. This inevitability is the reflection of the vast number of cells in the retina. An error in just one of these cells is enough to start the development of a cancer.

Cavanee and his colleagues (1984) showed Knudson's theory to be entirely correct by using a test called loss of heterozygosity (explained below). The retinoblastoma (*Rb*) gene discovery introduced a category of cancer genes initially called anti-oncogenes but now described as tumour suppressor genes. The function of these genes is not to prevent cancer (just as proto-oncogenes do not exist to cause cancer), rather cancer is a by-product of the loss of both functioning genes. The work of Knudson and Cavanee pointed to the possible existence of other tumour suppressor genes. Where else to find them but in other hereditary cancers?

The next hereditary form of cancer to be investigated was one known as familial adenomatous polyposis (FAP), which affects the colon and rectum (large intestine). Like retinoblastoma, this condition also runs in families as a dominant trait. Since an affected individual with a dominantly inherited condition carries one normal and one mutated gene, but can pass only one of these down to a child, each child has a fifty–fifty chance of receiving the mutated gene. In FAP, the development of many hundreds if not thousands of small mushroom-like polyps in the lining of the bowel begins in the teenage years of an affected individual. One or often more of these precancerous polyps or adenomas will inevitably develop into a cancer by the time the individual reaches the age of 40. This illustrates two general features of hereditary cancer: affected subjects are young, and they often develop multiple cancers.

The gene responsible for causing FAP was initially tracked down by a process called linkage analysis. The background to linkage is given in Chapter 27 but can be explained for the present purposes by the following analogy. It might become apparent in a cancer-prone family (this analogy is not true but explains the point) that all those who developed cancer had blue eyes. It would only be natural to assume some sort of connection. Then there might be another family in which many members were developing the same type of cancer, yet in the second family all the affected members were brown-eyed. This would indicate that eye colour was not causing the cancer, but that the gene determining eye colour (which is an inherited characteristic) always happened to be inherited in a pattern precisely fitting that of cancer development. The finding could be confirmed repeatedly in additional families until the odds against coincidence were astronomical, say one in a million (one in 10^6). Geneticists then convert this probability into a logarithm of the odds (LOD) score. 10^6 becomes a LOD score of 6. The test would not only prove that the cancer, like eye colour, was inherited, but would also show that the gene responsible for eye colour was on the same chromosome and very close to the gene causing cancer. In other words, the genes would be 'linked'. The fact of genetic recombination during the process of meiosis (see Chapter 27) provides linkage data which allows the distance between genetic loci to be measured.

To demonstrate linkage one needs to 'follow' genetic material through successive family generations. Such gene tracking is achieved with genetic markers that allow maternal and paternal DNA to be distinguished (since eye colour cannot be used in practice). Much of the DNA in chromosomes has no known function. Unlike junk mail, however, this DNA can be put to good use by the geneticist. Because it is junk, the non-coding DNA may accumulate mutations that are harmless. This accumulation leads to genetic variation (polymorphism) between individuals. And within one individual there will be variation between the maternal and paternal junk mail. How can this variation be detected? The tracking of linked genetic loci changed from wishful thinking to reality with the development of recombinant DNA technology, specifically Southern blotting and polymerase chain reaction based methods. Southern blotting will be considered first as it was the technique that resulted in the initial breakthroughs.

The variability between maternal and paternal junk DNA means that sites where DNA can be 'cut' with DNA cutting enzymes will vary. These enzymes are called restriction enzymes because they cut DNA only at restricted sites comprising specific base sequences. A single strand of DNA with a radioactive label will bind to a complementary sequence in both the maternal and paternal DNA. The DNA will have been extracted from millions of cells and so there will be millions of copies of the sequence of interest. The restriction enzyme then cuts the DNA into short lengths. However, the cutting sites or maternal and paternal DNA will differ and so the lengths of DNA bound to the probe will also differ. We can now imagine multiple bits of DNA, but of only two lengths only. The shorter lengths will travel faster than the longer ones when they are suspended in a gel through which a current is passed (electrophoresis). The difference is detected as the different movement of bands of DNA, still carrying the radioactive probe. In order to see the signal from the radioactive probe, the DNA must be 'blotted' from the gel onto paper. Since the technique was invented by Southern (1975) it is called a Southern blot. (There are also Northern blots for RNA and Western blots for protein—a sort of biochemical joke.)

The variability (polymorphism) in DNA that can be exploited by cutting DNA with restriction enzymes and tracking the different lengths as hereditary markers through family generations is encapsulated in the term 'restriction fragment length polymorphism (RFLP)' (Botstein et al., 1980). RFLPs exist for each chromosome and can be tracked through a family over and over again until a particular pattern of inheritance happens to coincide exactly with the inheritance of a (linked) gene responsible for an inherited disease. The demonstration of such linkage establishes, as explained above, that the disease is inherited and that the causative gene is not only on the same chromosome but very close to the RFLP. If one is lucky, however, one may know where to look to find linkage. In dividing cells chromosomes are large enough to be seen, and the technique of visualising chromosomes (called karyotyping) may indicate an obvious structural abnormality of one particular chromosome. In the case of the precancerous disorder familial adenomatous polyposis (FAP) (to which we now return), Herrera et al. (1986) demonstrated a large deletion in chromosome 5 of a man with FAP. Just a coincidence? Picking up on this clue, Bodmer et al. (1987) demonstrated linkage of FAP to chromosome 5, but it took four more years of positional cloning to pinpoint the gene termed *APC* (for adenomatous polyposis coli) and determine its exact structure. Even now, the function of *APC* is still being elucidated in full.

There is another very interesting side to the story of *APC*. As noted above, tumour suppressor genes contribute to the development of cancer when both copies are inactivated. Mutation may inactivate a tumour suppressor gene, but mutations are uncommon when DNA repair mechanisms are operating properly. It would clearly be somewhat of a coincidence for a mutation to inactivate a tumour suppressor gene in a particular normal cell, and then for the remaining normal (or wild type) copy of the same gene in the same cell (out of a total of about 100,000 genes) to be inactivated later by another mutation. Yet there is an alternative way of inactivating a gene without changing its structure by a mutation. This is by losing the gene altogether. During normal cell division (mitosis) it is not uncommon for an entire chromosome to go astray by a process known as non-disjunction. Suppose this quite common event occurs in a cell that already contains a mutated tumour suppressor gene. The chromosome that is lost may be the one that carries the normal gene. The result will be two copies of the mutated gene and no normal genes (Fig. 30). It is possible to prove that this has occurred within an established cancer by comparing the DNA in the cancer with the normal DNA from the individual with the cancer. One simply studies RFLPs (see above) within the chromosome known to carry the gene. There is the proviso that the RFLPs should be able to distinguish between the maternally- and paternally-derived DNA present in normal tissues. If one or other chromosome is missing in the cancer, the RFLP signal from that chromosome will not be detected in the cancer DNA (yet it is present in the normal DNA from the same individual). This is described as loss of heterozygosity (LOH), the term heterozygosity simply meaning that the maternal and paternal DNA is different. In the cancer, the ability to demonstrate this difference is lost. This is the test that Cavanee et al. (1984) used to prove that the *Rb* gene was a tumour suppressor gene (see above). LOH can also be demonstrated using PCR (see below).

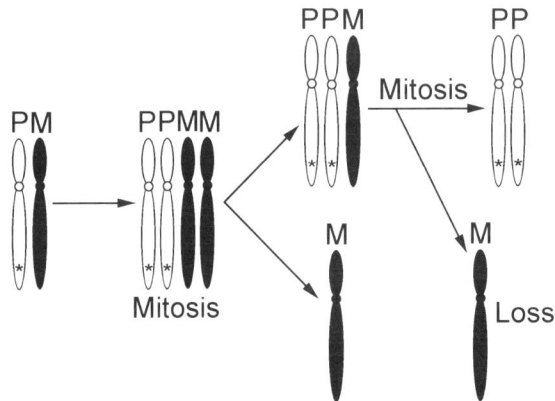

Figure 30 Mitotic non-disjunction. One of a pair of chromosomes (paternal = P) carries a mutation in the long arm. Non-disjunction occurs during mitosis. Three copies of the chromosome end up in one daughter cell and one in the other (may not be viable). At a second mitotic division, the maternal chromosome (M) carrying the wild type copy of the gene is lost. The resulting daughter cell now has two mutated genes.

Solomon et al. (1984) studied cancers from subjects with the hereditary disorder FAP, and were able to demonstrate the loss of chromosome 5 and particularly the region of chromosome 5 where the *APC* gene was located. This established the fact that *APC* was a tumour suppressor gene. It should be explained that it is not possible to demonstrate LOH unless it is present in a large clone of cells (all derived from a single cell). If LOH is limited to a small group of normal cells, the DNA signal will be too weak to be picked up. For LOH to be found throughout a large clonal population (such as a cancer) it must be providing some form of 'evolutionary' growth advantage. This may be described as the removal of the handbrake function of the normal copy of the tumour suppressor gene when the footbrake function of the other copy has been previously inactivated by a mutation. With both brakes not functioning, there is loss of control of cell proliferation.

Solomon et al. (1987) also showed loss of chromosome 5 in the common or non-inherited type of colorectal cancer. This was a crucial observation because it established the role of tumour suppressor genes in a common form of non-inherited cancer. It also showed how other types of tumour suppressor gene could be identified. One merely had to take a series of cancers of one type and see if particular chromosomes were lost on a consistent basis. If this were so, one could surmise that a tumour suppressor gene would be located on that chromosome. This approach has proved to be highly successful in colorectal and other types of cancer, and many tumour suppressor genes are now known to exist. Some such as *p53* have been found to play a role in many different types of cancer. Others are more restricted in their distribution amongst the various types of cancer.

MULTISTEP THEORY

Cancer is the end result of not one or two but many genetic alterations occurring in a distinct stepwise process. Each mutation (or gene loss) gives rise to a new subclone of daughter cells. One of these cells will in turn develop a mutation, and the altered cell may give rise to a further subclone and so on. The first steps may not lead to the development of a cancer but to a precancerous lesion (such as an adenoma in the case of the colorectum). Vogelstein et al. (1998) suggested that the development of a precancerous colorectal adenoma would require a particular sequence of genetic changes implicating at least three tumour suppressor genes: *APC* (early step), *DCC* (late step) and *p53* (late step), and an oncogene called *K-ras* (intermediate step). Tumour suppressor genes have already been likened to failed brakes that would allow a car to crash. Oncogenes act more like accelerators. The combination is clearly a recipe for disaster.

The mechanism underlying the pathogenesis of all cancers is an alteration of genetic material. But what is the cause of this alteration? In a small proportion of cancers, perhaps 5%, a key genetic mutation is inherited. In an individual carrying such a gene, every single cell is already one step towards becoming cancerous. This explains why inherited cancers occur at a relatively young age and are often multiple. Most genetic damage is acquired. The first step is DNA modification or damage caused by background ionising (cosmic or radon) or ultraviolet radiation or mutagenic chemicals. This may in turn lead to permanent genetic mutation as the damaged DNA is not repaired but is used as a template for DNA replication. Each time a chromosome is duplicated prior to cell division, a sequence of around one hundred million bases will need to be assembled in the correct order and within a time frame of a few hours. This provides many opportunities for error, and it is surprising that they are not more common. In fact errors must occur quite frequently, but are picked up by special proof-reading proteins which detect the mistake, cut it out and paste in the correct base sequence. As our cells age, this proofreading system becomes less effective and/or is itself inactivated by mutation. This leads us to consider the third main category of cancer genes.

DNA REPAIR GENES AND HYPERMUTABILITY

Conceivably mutations could inactivate the very genes that detect and repair mutations in other genes. This would allow mutations in cancer-causing genes to accumulate rapidly, a state of hypermutability. A long-established clinical model for this premise is provided by xeroderma pigmentosum, a rare autosomal dominant condition characterised by defective nucleotide excision repair. Affected individuals are extremely sensitive to ultraviolet light and develop multiple skin tumours at a young age.

It is now known that another type of DNA repair plays a much greater role in carcinogenesis. Before proceeding further, we need to return to the junk mail DNA. These areas of non-coding DNA (called microsatellites) often contain repetitive runs of bases (A, T, G and C; see Chapter 27) in which a single base, a pair or a triplet is repeated several times. The number of repeats, and therefore the length of these sequences, often varies between individuals. This variability forms the basis of the unique DNA fingerprint that characterises each individual, and which has proved so valuable in forensic science, evolutionary research and anthropology as well as clinical genetics. The easiest way to study this type of variation is by the powerful technique known as polymerase chain reaction (PCR) (Fig. 31). Finding a genetic sequence within the genome is harder than finding a needle in a haystack. If the genetic sequence is known, the PCR method can create a haystack made of needles by amplifying the sequence of interest an unlimited number of times. It is basically a method of

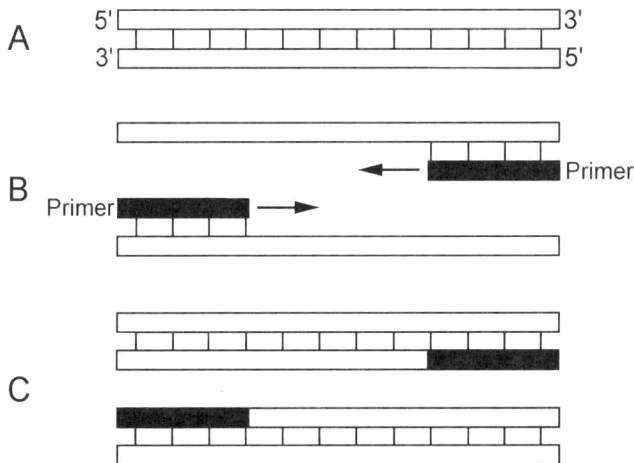

Figure 31 Polymerase chain reaction (PCR). Specific lengths of DNA can be replicated in the laboratory using primer sets. A: Target DNA sequence for amplification. B: Primers attached to denatured strands of DNA (by heating). C: Primers extend, thereby replicating the target DNA. This is again denatured and the cycle is repeated.

replicating DNA in the laboratory using the enzyme DNA polymerase that is employed by the cell for the same purpose (Saiki et al., 1988). This also provides the favoured approach for linkage studies and demonstration of LOH (Fig. 32). The PCR method also has multiple diagnostic uses for the histopathologist (Pan et al., 1995).

Two groups of researchers showed that innumerable mutations could be detected in the microsatellite regions of DNA obtained from about 15% of colorectal cancers, but not in the remainder (Ionov et al., 1993; Thibodeau et al., 1993). This meant that cancer DNA had a completely different DNA fingerprint from the normal DNA of the same individual (as though the cancer had literally become a new individual). This finding also applied to a form of hereditary colorectal cancer which is quite different from FAP in that it lacks the presence of multiple adenomas (Aaltonen et al., 1993), and which is described as hereditary non-polyposis colorectal cancer (HNPCC). Meanwhile, molecular biologists studying DNA repair genes in yeast (who would have thought this would turn out to have any direct relevance to man?) showed that mutations in these genes led to microsatellite mutations in yeast DNA. This group went on to suggest that similar genes in humans could be responsible for causing HNPCC (Strand et al., 1993). This principle of working out the function of a gene in a non-human species (bacterium, yeast, or the fruit fly *Drosophila*, for example) and appreciating that the same gene (or a near likeness) could be a candidate for a disease-causing gene in humans has led to the recognition of several cancer genes.

At the same time, a collaborative effort involving two large HNPCC families and researchers in the USA, Finland, Canada and New Zealand published a linkage study showing the location of a gene for HNPCC on chromosome 2 (Peltomäki et al., 1993). It took only a few months of positional cloning to find a gene in this region of chromosome 2 that was indeed similar to a yeast DNA repair gene called *MSH2*. A mutation of this gene involving a single base was found in a large New Zealand family, affecting every single member with colorectal cancer, but exempting the older generations, who were free of the cancer (Leach *et al.*, 1993). This perfect segregation of the mutation with cancer development proved beyond doubt that the candidate DNA repair gene was the inherited cause of cancer in this family. The DNA repair genes (an entire family of what are now termed specifically DNA mismatch repair genes) have been implicated not only in the inherited condition HNPCC but also in the 15%

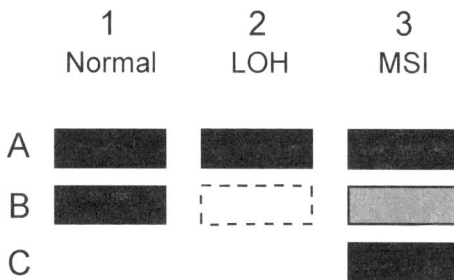

Figure 32 Two principal types of genetic change seen in tumour DNA following microsatellite region analysis by PCR. The normal lane (1) shows two alleles of maternal and paternal origin. The LOH lane (2) shows loss of heterozygosity or loss of the allele B. The MSI lane (3) shows a lane deletion (mutation) affecting allele B. The amount of allele B is reduced (residual amounts in non-mutated DNA), whereas an extra band C appears.

of non-familial colorectal cancers showing multiple microsatellite mutations. DNA repair genes function as tumour suppressor genes inasmuch as both copies must be inactivated or lost to bring about cancer development. The year of the DNA mismatch repair gene was 1993.

In this chapter, three types of hereditary cancer have been discussed, one of the eye and two of the large intestine, since these led to the recognition of two of the three major classes of cancer gene. The study of hereditary cancers of the breast, ovary, stomach, kidney, prostate, skin and endocrine organs has led to the discovery of many more cancer genes since 1993. However, all of these genes have fallen into the categories of oncogenes (*RET, MET*), tumour suppressor genes (*APC, TP53, VHL, NF1, NF2, INK4, CDK4, PTC* and *cadherin*) and DNA repair genes (*hMSH2, hMSH6, hMLH1, hPMS1, hPMS2, BRCA1-2*) (Caldas & Ponder, 1997). The same genes are often (but not always) responsible for both the inherited and the non-inherited cancers arising in a particular organ. The main exceptions are the DNA repair genes which operate in hereditary cancers but less frequently in non-familial cancers.

PROMOTING AGENTS AND EPIGENETIC MECHANISMS IN CARCINOGENESIS

The generation of a cancer would appear to be the culmination of a sequence of irreversible genomic changes—a permanent reprogramming of the instructional machinery of the cell. This stark view leaves us with little room for therapeutic manoeuvre other than ablation by surgery or chemoradiotherapy. While the concept of cancer as a genetic disease is fundamentally correct, there are several important caveats with exciting therapeutic implications.

Promoting agents

It has long been known that a single mutagen will cause cancer if given in sufficient dose. In practice humans are not exposed to high concentrations of carcinogens. A low mutagenic dose, on the other hand, may initiate the process of carcinogenesis by priming the target tissue with mutations. The effect of promoting agents is not to cause additional mutations by a direct mechanism, but to provide conditions that favour the proliferation of initiated cells. Examples are the phorbol esters which serve as analogues of the powerful signalling molecule diacylglycerol (see page 71).

A genetic mutation is perceived as a qualitative and final alteration, but the downstream effects on cell function are quantitative, and therefore either reversible or capable of being bypassed through the activation of appropriate molecular pathways. A number of agents are known to be anti-promotional and potentially capable of preventing cancer (Hong & Sporn, 1997). Administration of the non-steroidal anti-inflammatory drug sulindac results in regression of adenomas in the condition FAP (see above). The abnormal growth of adenomas in FAP is explained by prostaglandin mediated down-regulation of apoptosis. The enzyme cyclooxygenase, which converts arachidonic acid to prostaglandin G_2 (see page 74), is upregulated in adenomatous cells and sulindac happens to block the activity of this enzyme. Vitamin E and retinoic acid also appear to check the growth of initiated cells—prostate cancer in the case of vitamin E, and of several types of cancer in the case of retinoic acid. Retinoic acid may even cause certain established cancers (e.g. promyelocytic leukemia) to regress.

Altered methylation

Apart from the possibilities of bypassing the effects of mutated cancer genes, there is firm evidence that abnormal methylation of DNA (at islands rich in CpG sequences) plays a critical epigenetic role in the evolution of cancer. Hypomethylation results in chromosomal instability, while several tumour suppressor genes (E-cadherin, *p16, ptc, Rb, VHL, WT1* and *hMLH1*) can be inactivated by hypermethylation of the promoter region (as well as by mutation or LOH). The normal function of methylation is unclear but may be related to the need to suppress 'parasitic' DNA sequences that are inadvertently introduced into a gene during DNA replication. Once the mechanism of hypermethylation is fully elucidated, the possibility of preventing or reversing this phenomenon should have a major impact on cancer management (Baylin et al., 1998).

It can now be stated without a shadow of doubt that cancer is a disease resulting from the alteration of the genetic machinery of a cell, whether this be acquired or inherited. This understanding began in 1953 with the demonstration by Watson and Crick of the structure of the gene, and culminated forty years later with the recognition of three main classes of cancer gene. The list of cancer genes is not complete and we have yet to explain fully the normal function of these genes and how normal function is subverted in the cancer cell. Nevertheless, an understanding of the underlying principles is firmly in place, and powerful molecular techniques for building upon this knowledge are available. Completion of the story is now just a matter of time.

Additional aspects of cancer genetics, specifically the interface between anatomical pathology and genetics, are considered in Chapter 27.

REFERENCES

Aaltonen, L.A., Peltomäki, P., Leach, F.S., Sistonen, P., Pylkkänen, L., Mecklin, J.P., Järvinen, H., Powell, S.M., Jen, J. & Hamilton, S.R. et al. (1993) Clues to the pathogenesis of familial colorectal cancer. *Science,* **260**, 812–816.

Baltimore, D. (1970) Viral RNA-dependent DNA polymerase. *Nature,* **226**, 1209–1211.

Baylin, S.B., Herman, J.G., Graff, J.R., Vertino, P.M. & Issa, J.P. (1998) Alterations in DNA methylation: a fundamental aspect of neoplasia. *Adv Cancer Res,* **72**, 141–196.

Bodmer, W.F., Bailey, C.J., Bodmer, J., Bussey, H.J.R., Ellis, A., Gorman, P., Lucibello, F.C., Murday, F.A., Rider, S.H., Scambler, P., Sheer, D., Solomon, E. & Spurr, N. (1987) Localization of the gene for familial adenomatous polyposis on chromosome 5. *Nature,* **328**, 614 616.

Botstein, D., White, R.L., Skolnick, M. & Davis, R.W. (1980) Construction of a genetic linkage map in man using restriction fragment length polymorphisms. *Am J Hum Genet,* **32**, 314–331.

Caldas, C. & Ponder, B.A.J. (1997) Cancer genes and molecular oncology in the clinic. *Lancet,* **349**(suppl II), 16–18.

Cavance, W.K., Dryja, T.P., Phillips, R.A., Rapaport, J.M., Petersen, R., Albert, D.H. & Bruns, G.A. (1984) Homozygosity of the retinoblastoma gene on chromosome 13. *New Engl J Med,* **310**, 550–553.

Herrera, L., Kakati, Gibas, L., Pietrzak, E. & Sandberg, A.A. (1986) Gardner syndrome in a man with an interstitial deletion of 5q. *Am J Med Genet,* **25**, 473–476.

Hong, W.K. & Sporn, B.M. (1997) Recent advances in the chemoprevention of cancer. *Science,* **278**, 1073–1077.

Ionov, Y.M., Peinado, A., Malkhosyan, S., Shibata, D. & Perucho, M. (1993) Ubiquitous somatic mutations in simple repeated sequences reveal a new mechanism for colonic carcinogenesis. *Nature*, **363**, 558–561.

Knudson, A.G. (1971) Mutation and cancer: statistical study of retinoblastoma. *Proc Natl Acad Sci USA,* **68**, 820–823.

Leach, F.S., Nicolaides, N.C., Papadopoulos, N., Liu, B., Jen, J., Parsons, P., Peltomäki, P., Sistonen, P., Aaltonen, L.A. & Nystrom-Lahti, M., et al. (1993) Mutations of a *mut*S homolog in hereditary nonpolyposis colorectal cancer. *Cell*, **75**, 1215–1225.

Pan, L.X., Diss, T.C. & Isaacson, P.G. (1995) The polymerase chain reaction in histopathology. *Histopathology*, **26**, 201–217.

Peltomäki, P., Aaltonen, L.A., Sistonen, P., Pylkkänen, L., Mecklin, J.P., Järvinen, H., Green, J.S., Jass, J.R., Weber, J.L. & Leach, F.S., et al. (1993) Genetic mapping of a locus predisposing to human colorectal cancer. *Science*, **260**, 810–812.

Saiki, R.K., Gelfand, D.H., Stoffel, S., Scharf, S.J., Higuchi, R., Horn, G.T., Mullis, K.B. & Erlich, H.A. (1988) Primer-detected enzymatic amplification of DNA with a thermostable polymerase. *Science*, **239**, 487–491.

Sambrook, J., Westphal, H., Srinivasan, R. & Dulbecco, R. (1968) The integrated state of viral DNA in SV40-transformed cells. *Proc Natl Acad Sci USA,* **60**, 1288–1295.

Solomon, E., Voss, R., Hall, V., Bodmer, W.F., Jass, J.R., Jeffreys, A.J., Lucibello, F.C., Patel, I. & Rider, S.H. (1987) Chromosome 5 allele loss in human colorectal carcinomas. *Nature,* **328**, 616–619.

Southern, E.M. (1975) Detection of specific sequences among DNA fragments separated by gel electrophoresis. *J Mol Biol,* **98**, 503–517.

Strand, M., Prolla, T.A., Liskay, R.M. & Petes, T. (1993) Destabilisation of tracts of simple repetitive DNA in yeast by mutation affecting DNA mismatch repair. *Nature*, **365**, 274–276.

Temin, H.M. & Mizutani, S. (1970) Viral RNA-dependent DNA polymerase. *Nature,* **226**, 1211–1213.

Vogelstein, B., Fearon, E.R., Hamilton, S.R., Kern, S.E., Preisinger, A.C., Leppert, M., Nakamura, Y., White, R., Smits, A.M.M. & Bos, J.L. (1988) Genetic alterations during colorectal-tumour development. *New Engl J Med*, **319**, 525–532.

24

CLONALITY, GROWTH AND
SPREAD OF CANCER

*That a tumour, one's own tumour, the destructive tumour which has mangled
one's whole life should suddenly drain away, dry up and die by itself?*

Alexander Solzhenitsyn *(Cancer Ward)*

How does a cancer spread?

CLONALITY

Clonality implies that cancer, which may comprise thousands of millions of cells, originates
from a single cell. The ability of a single cell to give rise to large numbers of cells is not limited
to cancer. Normal tissues include a permanent set of stem cells (see Chapter 16). These are like
an ancestor from the past who is continually giving birth to new children, grandchildren and
great grandchildren; the descendants will pass away but the ancestor is immortal. A cancer
can be traced back to an 'immortal' stem cell rather than to a descendant that is committed to
a limited lifespan. However, most of the cells in a cancer will have a limited lifespan. In fact
when one attempts to grow cells from a cancer in a laboratory, they usually die within a short
period. Occasionally one cell may survive to form a 'cell line' that can be used for further
experiments. Such a cell would be the malignant equivalent of a normal stem cell.

The reason why a neoplasm must ultimately be derived from a stem cell is that the stepwise
accumulation of genetic errors takes time, and only stem cells persist long enough to sustain
the required number of mutational 'hits'. Yet the final transforming mutation may affect a
daughter cell rather than the stem cell itself. There are four lines of argument that would
support this contention: (1) that stem cells divide slowly, more slowly than their daughters,
(2) that daughter cells are more numerous than stem cells and therefore represent a larger
target population, (3) that hits within different daughter cell generations provide an explanation for different grades of differentiation within early neoplasms, and (4) that neoplastic
crypts have been shown to bud from the side of normal crypts in colonic mucosa (Fig. 33)
(Nakamura & Iino, 1984). However, the origin of early adenoma from a daughter cell must
involve the retention or acquisition of stem cell propertics by the transformed daughter cells.

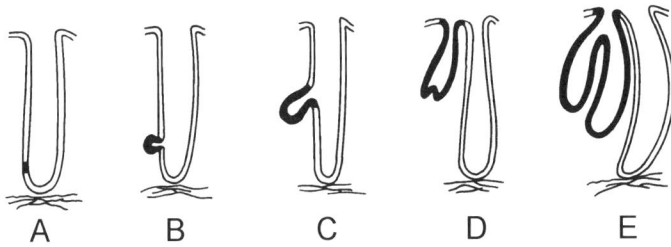

Figure 33 Origin of adenoma from a single colorectal crypt. A: Cell is transformed. B: Adenomatous bud is formed as an outgrowth of the parent crypt. C: Bud forms tubule as it migrates upwards. D: Adenomatous tubule opens onto surface epithelium and fission begins. E: Microadenoma comprising two neoplastic crypts. This will grow by further crypt fission.

The adenoma may transform into a carcinoma subsequently, the adenoma—carcinoma sequence. *De novo* cancers (arising directly from morphologically normal-appearing epithelium) may arise when the final transforming hit implicates a stem cell.

The clonal nature of neoplasm can be demonstrated in a number of ways. Like many endocrine glands, the anterior pituitary comprises multiple glands in one. With the use of a dual stain (periodic acid Schiff/Orange G), one can see that the gland comprises intermingled cells which are either periodic acid Schiff positive (magenta) or exclusively Orange G positive. A neoplasm of the anterior pituitary, however, may be exclusively periodic acid Schiff positive (secreting the hormone ACTH) or Orange G positive (secreting growth hormone and prolactin), but not positive using both techniques. Similarly, normal B lymphocytes secrete either kappa or lambda light chains whereas a neoplasm of B lymphocytes produces a light chain of one class only. It could be argued that the neoplastic process is occurring within cells of one type only, but is still polyclonal with respect to cells of that type.

A more definitive proof of clonality is achieved by examining a single population of cells in which it is possible to differentiate two classes of cell on the basis of an entirely random feature that cannot be linked to the neoplastic process. In females only one or the other X chromosome is active within cells. The other takes the form of a condensation of chromatin that is visible on the inner side of the nuclear membrane as a Barr body (the latter is found only in cells of female origin and can be used to determine gender). Lyon suggested that one or the other X chromosome would be inactivated on a random and fifty–fifty basis. In a female, one X chromosome is paternally derived and the other is maternally derived. There will be multiple differences between the two chromosomes at the genetic level (polymorphism). For example, the gene coding for the enzyme glucose 6 phosphate dehydrogenase (G6PD) resides on the X chromosome. One form of G6PD is very common (G6PDA), but a variant (G6PDB) is mainly limited to certain races, notably blacks. A black female will be informative for the demonstration of clonality if her maternally- and paternally- derived G6PD happens to include isozymes A and B but not AA or BB. If a biochemical or histochemical technique is applied in order to distinguish A and B (e.g. by employing a monoclonal antibody which recognises one type only), then clonality will be proven if the neoplastic population comprises cells of one type in background of cells of both types (Fig. 34).

Molecular technology provides less awkward ways of showing clonality. Gene rearrangement is the basis of the uniqueness of cells of the immune system (genes coding for the

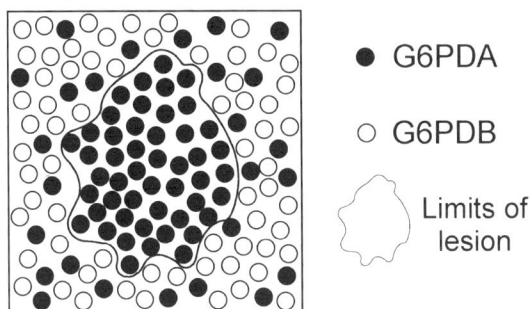

Figure 34 Clonal lesion arising within a polyclonal background

receptors of T cells or immunoglobulins of B cells) (page 85). One particular unique immune cell will not stand out from all the others when rearranged genes are probed. However, in a lymphoid neoplasm the amount of rearranged DNA will be increased to detectable levels as a result of clonal expansion. Similarly, a genetic mutation will be detectable if it implicates a clone of sufficient size. For example, if the mutation initiated the neoplastic process then it will be present in all parts of the neoplasm. However, one may also be able to demonstrate clonality within a normal-appearing cell population if the mutation has occurred in an immortal (or near-immortal) stem cell that supports a clonal patch. In other words, clonality *per se* is not equivalent to neoplasia, even when its demonstration rests on the finding of a mutated gene known to be implicated in carcinogenesis.

POLYCLONALITY

Although it is widely accepted that cancers are clonal, bona fide benign neoplasms can be polyclonal. How can this be? The paradox arises in rare situations when an individual (or genetically engineered animal) carries a germline mutation that predisposes them to the development of multiple neoplasms. This was first shown in a patient with familial adenomatous polyposis (FAP) who also happened to have an unrelated chromosomal mosaicism (XO/XY). A proportion of this individual's stem cells was XO and the remainder XY. If an adenoma were clonal either all or none of its cells would carry a Y chromosome. In fact, adenomas were found to be patchwork or polyclonal in this regard (Novelli et al., 1996). It would seem that the proximity of two or more small clones (which individually might remain microscopic) leads to mutual growth promotion and the development of a visible polyp (adenoma). It should be stressed that polyclonality is a form of collision of independent clones that appears to be mutually advantageous to further growth. It is the exception rather than the rule.

Polyclonality is different from subclonal generation. Within a neoplasm, and perhaps especially during early neoplastic evolution, new mutations are arising constantly. Those conferring a growth advantage will lead to the generation of subclones. One of these will eventually acquire malignant potential and destroy the less aggressive subclones that were its predecessors, just as a newly evolved species may compete with and destroy its closest rivals (Fig. 35).

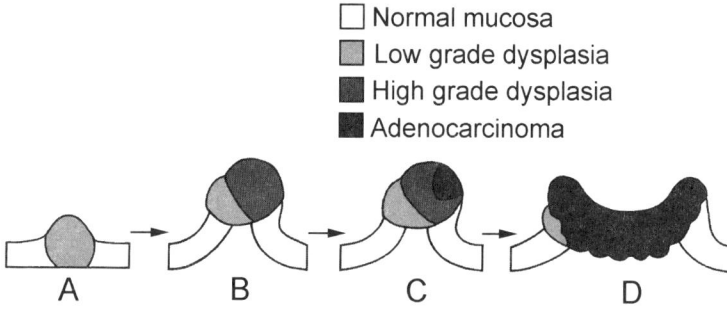

Figure 35 Adenoma to carcinoma sequence (e.g. occurring within colorectal mucosa). A: Small adenoma. B: More rapidly growing subclone showing high grade dysplasia. C: Development of a malignant subclone. D: Growth of malignant subclone which has ulcerated and destroyed all but a fraction of the original adenoma.

FIELD CHANGE

There is, however, a contradictory view to the clonal theory which states that cancer begins in an area of 'field change'. It is certainly true that the tissues surrounding a cancer may not be entirely normal. Cancers often arise in organs that have been altered by longstanding inflammation associated with numerous cycles of damage and repair. Examples would be inflammation of the stomach (chronic gastritis), colon (ulcerative colitis), liver (cirrhosis) and sunlight-exposed skin. Other organs prone to cancer may not be common sites of inflammation but may show various forms of architectural disorganisation (hyperplasia) that are likely to be related to an abnormal hormonal responsiveness (e.g. the breast and prostate). It should be emphasised that the risk of cancer in patients with the above background conditions is increased by only a small factor over and above the general population. These examples indicate that relatively minor but repeated and longstanding types of injury will increase the likelihood of genetic mutations. Indeed tissues with rapid cellular turnover that are continuously exposed to environmental factors (e.g. the skin, gut, bronchi of lung) may be peppered with cells containing mutations (Ogden & Hall, 1997). Modern techniques allow these mutations to be demonstrated with relative ease. Most will be completely harmless, whereas a minority may progress further.

Generally speaking, therefore, any 'field change' surrounding a cancer is not a continuous sheet of abnormal cells, but an area containing focal alterations that are of little or no individual significance, but together may carry a small risk to the patient (more like a field of blighted seeds). This would explain why a patient may develop over time two or more independent cancers in the same organ or tissue (genetic predisposition may also account for this; see Chapter 23). This should be distinguished from recurrence of the same cancer due to incomplete excision by the surgeon.

METASTASIS

The property of spread underlies the lethality of cancer. The full menace of cancer is realised when it spreads beyond its site of origin and sets up colonies in distant organs. Once metastasis occurs, treatment is unlikely to be curative. What is the cause of the seemingly relentless spread of cancer? We can turn this question around and ask why normal cells do not spread. In fact single cells do spread, whether they be single-celled organisms such as amoebae or the white blood cells of higher organisms. Cells organised into tissues do not spread because they are anchored to each other and to connective tissue elements by means of adhesion molecules (page 104). In some cancers, the genes encoding adhesion molecules are mutated and cell-to-cell adhesion breaks down (Becker et al., 1997). Single, highly infiltrative signet ring cells are thus produced (page 105). It is not necessary for a cancer to become single celled for invasion to occur. The uncontrolled growth of a mass of cells will tend to induce invasion by a simple pressure effect. This will be facilitated by the abnormal production of proteolytic enzymes by the cancer cells (van der Burg et al., 1996) and by the surrounding stroma (Nielsen et al., 1996). Groups of cancer cells will tend to travel by routes offering the least resistance, seeking out potential spaces beneath the sheaths that surround nerves or following the paths already trodden by the ramifying vasculature of the body. Angiogenesis, or the development of a tumour microvasculature, is a critical step, providing not only essential nutrients but also an escape route for malignant cells (Folkman & D'Amore, 1996).

Mechanisms

Once cancer cells penetrate into the lumen (central cavity) of a vessel they can travel large distances with relative ease (Willis, 1952). Two types of vessel may be invaded: lymphatics and veins. One function of the lymphatic system is to prevent tissue swelling by draining excess fluid from the spaces between cells, returning it to the blood. The passage of fluid is interrupted by the presence of lymph nodes, whose principal function is to monitor invasion by micro-organisms and mount an appropriate immune response. Cancer cells may be trapped in lymph nodes, where they form secondary deposits. Eventually some cells will break away and continue along the lymphatic chain, spreading from node to node. It is for this reason that cancer surgery removes not only the main tumour but also the draining lymph nodes which may have succeeded in limiting the extent of spread. Once cancer has spread to lymph nodes, the chances of cure are reduced. By setting up colonies in lymph nodes the cancer has indicated it is capable of metastasis.

Distant spread occurs in a more direct way when cancer cells enter the venous system. Cancer of the stomach, pancreas or bowel, for example, may then spread directly to the liver. From the liver, cancer cells may re-enter the circulation to reach the lung. Cancer cells originating from other sites will be held up in the microcirculation of the lung and form secondary deposits. The liver and lung are common sites for the first wave of secondary cancer deposits. From the lung, cancer cells will pass to the left side of the heart to be pumped to all the tissues of the body (Weiss et al., 1986).

The fact that cancer cells have entered the circulatory system does not mean that colonisation of distant sites is inevitable. The blood contains white blood cells, antibodies and proteins that will entrap and destroy cancer cells. Furthermore, the circulation is a closed system filled with rapidly flowing blood. To reach other organs, cancer cells must not only evade the natural defences in the blood, but must adhere to the endothelial cells lining vessels and squeeze their way through these tightly apposed cells. This will require the acquisition of new adhesion molecules and the capacity for amoeboid movement. Once outside a vessel, the cancer cell must be able to obtain nourishment and grow to form a colony in an environment quite different from the tissue of its origin.

Metastatic cancer cells have requirements about where they will and will not grow (Table 9). The liver is a popular site for most carcinomas and lymphomas but not for sarcomas. Sarcomas rarely metastasise to any sites other than the lungs. Bones are a common site of secondary spread for cancers of the breast, prostate, lung, kidney and thyroid. Lung, breast and kidney cancers may spread to the brain. Some organs or tissues are very rare sites for secondary cancer, for example the spleen, kidney and skeletal muscle. Malignant melanoma can spread to virtually any site in the body. These observations have led to the seed and soil hypothesis to explain metastasis. Both the seed (cancer cell) and soil (distant site) must have the required characteristics. Knowledge of where a cancer can and cannot spread is important for determining whether a tumour is primary or secondary and, if secondary, the likely primary source. Occasionally the primary source may regress before secondary disease becomes manifest. This is well documented for malignant melanoma and means that secondary deposits can sometimes appear in an apparently healthy patient without warning. In general, however, spread of cancer occurs as a late process, typically some years after the initial cancer diagnosis.

It is clear that a cancer cell must acquire multiple new characteristics if it is to establish distant colonies (Fidler, 1973). This in turn depends on the gradual and stepwise build-up of genetic changes that will govern each of the newly acquired properties of the cancer cell. This cannot occur in a few days. In some cases the transformation of a single initiated cell into a cancer with full metastatic potential may take many years, even decades. This forms the rationale for screening and early detection of cancer.

STAGING

As explained in Chapter 22, definitive treatment of a cancer generally depends not only on the diagnosis of malignancy but also on the type and grade. The clinician also needs to know that the growth is primary and not a colony that has spread from elsewhere. Knowledge of the

Table 9 Sites of metastases

Metastatic site	Carcinoma and Melanoma	Lymphoma	Sarcoma
Lymph nodes	+++	+++	+/-
Liver	+++	++	+
Body cavities	+++	+	-
Lung	++	+	+++
Brain	++	+	-
Bone marrow	++	+++	+/-
Adrenal	++	-	-
Spleen	+	++	-
Skin	+	++	-
Thyroid	+	+/-	-
Breast	+	+/-	+/-
Kidney	+/-	+	-
Heart	+/-	+/-	+/-
Skeletal muscle	+/-	+/-	-

extent of spread can be acquired by examination of the patient and through various imaging modalities. However, the most objective evidence regarding extent of local spread is obtained through the meticulous examination and dissection of a surgical specimen of cancer. This is described as pathological staging. The pathologist is also in a position to determine whether surgical excision successfully removed the entire growth, and to audit the technical proficiency of the procedure.

The approach to pathological staging is similar for all types of cancer and reflects the major routes of spread: local, lymphatic and venous. This translates into the widely used code of TNM. In this system T defines the extent of spread of the tumour, N stands for nodal (lymph node) involvement and M refers to metastatic disease. When a tumour is growing in a solid or homogenous organ, the extent of spread is defined objectively by measuring the maximum diameter of the growth. In such situations there is no reason why the cancer shouldn't expand equally in all directions, giving a roughly spherical mass, e.g. as applicable in breast cancer. When a cancer arises in the lining of a multilayered hollow tube such as the colon, local spread (T) is determined by depth of penetration through the various anatomical layers of the bowel wall. The human body contains a number of cavities, such as the peritoneal cavity in the abdomen and the pleural cavity within the thorax, which are lined by serous membranes. In the abdomen this membrane, the peritoneum, covers all the organs and provides the final barrier against spread in the case of a cancer arising in the lining of an organ such as the stomach or colon or within the ovary. The thin membrane nevertheless serves as a potent barrier to cancer spread (and to the spread of infection), but once breached the cancer cells can traverse the cavity and implant themselves widely. Such transperitoneal spread is often associated with seepage of fluid (ascites) into the abdominal cavity, which then becomes distended. Transperitoneal spread is given a separate T number code because of its serious portent (Shepherd et al., 1995). Nodal spread (N) is graded by the number of involved lymph nodes. Information on metastatic spread (M) requires clinical input and the diagnosis should ideally be confirmed by biopsy and microscopic examination. Nodules in sites such as the liver may closely resemble cancer macroscopically, yet be perfectly harmless. The bile duct hamartoma is an example of one such innocent hepatic lesion.

Since staging documents the extent of anatomical spread of cancer, it provides one of the most important guide to prognosis. Cancer that is localised to the site of origin and has not spread to lymph nodes draining the affected region is usually completely curable by surgery. Although cure is rarely achieved once cancer has spread widely, the recognition of distant spread is not always straightforward. A particular difficulty arises when cancer is scattered as microscopic groups of cells in such organs as the liver or bone marrow. Some cancers secrete chemicals (tumour markers) into the bloodstream. If these substances are detected in a blood sample after the surgical removal of the primary tumour, one may infer that spread has occurred to distant sites. However, small numbers of cancer cells may not be detectable. Sometimes bone scans and liver scans can pick up micrometastases, but these techniques are not reliable and provide no histologically verified proof of cancer.

PROGNOSTIC CLASSIFICATION

Reliance has to be placed on other prognostic factors and these will largely be based on the pathological examination of the specimen. The general approach has been to study very large groups of patients who have received treatment that was considered to be curative. The group is followed up for many years, during which time a subset will show evidence of recurrent disease in distant sites and succumb to the cancer. These distant sites were almost certainly colonised at the time of treatment, but the groups of malignant cells were then too small to be detected. Conversely the rest of the patients will be cancer-free— totally cured.

Such results have lead to the assessment of pathological features shown by such cancers which have distinguished the survivors from the non-survivors. Using a method called logistic regression analysis one is able to pinpoint features that lend independent information to this process of discrimination. These features may include the number of lymph nodes, the size or extent of spread, the grade (see Chapter 22), the presence of oestrogen receptors in the case of breast cancer and many other variables. By selecting from a comprehensive set of variables a subset of three or four that are important and easily reproducible for a particular type of cancer, one is able to derive reliable prognostic information. Such prognostic models have been developed for several types of cancer (Jass et al., 1987). Although this is certainly a worthwhile approach, it is very difficult to achieve a universally acceptable system that is clearly superior in the hands of all users. Furthermore, prognostic indices can only give estimates of probable outcomes for individual patients, such as a 95% certainty of cure, or a 5% certainty of cure. Nevertheless such guidance can be useful for individuals who would otherwise be planning for a life expectancy of 20 years.

REFERENCES

Becker, I. Becker, K.F., Rohrl, M.H., Minkus, G., Schutze, K. & Höfler, H. (1996) Single-cell mutation analysis of tumours from stained histologic slides. *Lab Invest,* **75**, 801–807.

Fidler, I.J. (1973) Selection of successive tumour lines for metastasis. *Nature,* **242**, 148–149.

Folkman, J. & D'Amore, P.A. (1996) Blood vessel formation: What is its molecular basis? *Cell,* **87**, 1153–1155.

Jass, J.R., Love, S.B. & Northover, J.M.A. (1987) A new prognostic classification of rectal cancer. *Lancet,* **i**, 1303–1306.

Nakamura, S. & Kino, I. (1984) Morphogenesis of minute adenomas in familial polyposis coli. *J Natl Cancer Inst,* **73**, 41–49.

Nielson, B.S., Sehested, M., Timshel, S., Pyke, C. & Dano, K. (1996) Messenger for urokinase plasminogen activator is expressed by myofibroblasts adjacent to cancer cells in human breast cancer. *Lab Invest,* **74**, 168–177.

Novelli, M.R., Williamson, J.A., Tomlinson, I.P.M., Elia, G., Hodgson, S.V., Talbot, I.G., Bodmer, W.F. & Wright, N.A. (1996) Polyclonal origin of colonic adenomas in an XO/XY patient with FAP. *Science,* **272**, 1187–1190.

Ogden, G.R. & Hall, P.A. (1997) Field change, clonality and early epithelial cancer. *J Pathol,* **181**, 127–129.

Shepherd, N.A., Baxter, K.J. & Love, S.B. (1995) Influence of local peritoneal involvement on pelvic recurrence and prognosis in rectal cancer. *J Clin Pathol,* **48**, 849–855.

van der Burg, M.E., Henzen-Logmans, S.C., Berns, E.M., van Putten, W.L., Klijn, J.G. & Foekens, J.A. (1996) Expression of urokinase-type plasminogen activator (UPA) and its inhibitor PAI-1 in benign, borderline, malignant primary and metastatic ovarian tumours. *Int J Cancer,* **69**, 475–479.

Weiss, L., Grundmann, E., Torhorst, J., Hartveit, F., Moberg, I., Eder, M., Fenoglio-Preiser, C.M., Napier, J., Horne, C.H. & Lopez, M.J., *et al.* (1986) Haematogenous metastatic patterns in colonic carcinoma: an analysis of 1541 necropsies. *J Pathol,* **150**, 195–203.

Willis, R.A. (1952) *The Spread of Tumours in the Human Body*. London: Butterworth and Co.

Further reading

Sobin, L.H. & Wittekind, Ch. (1997) *TNM Classification of Malignant Tumours*. New York: Wiley &Sons, Inc.

Vile, R.G. & Hart, I.R. (1995) The molecular basis of metastasis. In *Progress in Pathology*, volume 1, edited by N. Kirkham & P. Hall, pp. 133–150. Edinburgh: Churchill Livingstone.

25

EPITHELIAL PRECANCEROUS AND BORDERLINE LESIONS: DIAGNOSIS AND SCREENING

God does not play dice

Albert Einstein

What is a precancerous lesion?

BORDERLINE LESIONS

Over the years clinicians have come to expect clear-cut diagnoses from the anatomical pathologist. The historical reasons for this may be traced to the tradition of the clinicopathological conference. This expectation reaches its zenith in relation to cancer diagnosis; the patient either does or does not have cancer. The dividing line between cancer and non-cancer is not necessarily sharp. There are lesions that fall into a grey area by virtue of their uncertain status on the pathway of neoplastic progression. The term 'non-cancer' is used for such lesions because lesions on the benign side of the divide will not be normal. A genetically transformed cell may divide to form a lesion that is microscopically visible if not sufficiently large or protuberant so as to be felt or noticed. Such asymptomatic lesions may be detected through screening programs (such as those for breast cancer or cervical cancer), through increased awareness of the appearances of early cancer (such as malignant melanoma) or fortuitously by the pathologist examining a surgical specimen for another reason (such as in the case of an advanced cancer). If the neoplastic process is a continuum, where does one draw the line between cancer and non-cancer?

The classification of borderline lesions is one of the more controversial areas in tumour pathology. Consideration in this chapter will be limited to epithelial lesions. One may adopt a strictly laboratory-based approach using specific microscopic criteria alone to formulate a diagnosis. Alternatively, classifications may be influenced by clinical observations regarding the behaviour of a lesion. Common to both approaches is the key anatomical landmark used to distinguish epithelial pre-cancer (benign neoplasia) from cancer: the basement membrane.

DYSPLASIA

Neoplasia that has not transversed the basement membrane but is instead confined to the epithelial layer may either be flat or produce a visible mass. The diagnostic changes seen in both flat and protuberant neoplasms have been described as dysplasia and are recognised by a combination of altered architecture, impaired differentiation and, most importantly, cellular atypia. A cell is described as showing severe or high grade atypia when the appearances of its nucleus approach those of a cancer cell (see Chapter 21). Neoplastic tissue composed of such cells may be described as severe dysplasia, carcinoma-in-situ or high-grade intra-epithelial neoplasia (Fig. 36). The precise terminology varies for different anatomical sites, types of lesion and 'schools' of pathology. However, when no evidence of invasion can be demonstrated, pathologists are generally agreed that an unqualified diagnosis of cancer is unwarranted. For many, even the term carcinoma-in-situ carries an excessively aggressive connotation which could be misconstrued. At the other end of the spectrum, mild or low-grade epithelial dysplasia describes changes that are considered neoplastic but deviate minimally from the normal. The risk that a dysplastic lesion will progress to cancer increases proportionately to the grade of dysplasia. However, for an individual patient the magnitude of risk cannot be stated with any certainty.

The term dysplasia is associated with a number of practical difficulties. Its meaning varies in different pathological contexts. For example, it may be used to describe abnormal embryological development without neoplastic potential in organs such as the kidney. In the present context, dysplasia relates to a precancerous epithelial change falling short of malignancy (pre-invasive or benign neoplasia). Dysplasia may be mimicked by tissues undergoing repair or regeneration in response to a variety of inflammatory stimuli. This is a common problem in practice. Benign epithelial neoplasms show dysplasia by definition, but are classified according to the type of neoplasm (see Chapter 22). Small biopsies from the surface of a cancer may be underdiagnosed as dysplasia. In some tissues, for example breast and endometrium, dysplasia is manifested by a combination of epithelial overgrowth (hyperplasia) and cytological atypia. These lesions are usually described as hyperplasia with atypia rather than as dysplasia. In the cervix and prostate the term 'intra-epithelial neoplasia' is preferred to dysplasia. In short, the term dysplasia is subject to non-standardised use as well as abuse.

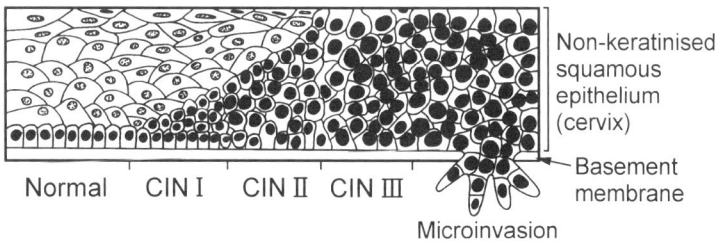

Figure 36 Progression through grades of cervical intra-epithelial neoplasia (CIN) to micro-invasion. There is replacement of regularly maturing squamous epithelium by atypical basal cells. The latter have proliferative capacity and show atypical nuclear features (enlargement and hyperchromatism).

Employed with care in the case of biopsies from the gastrointestinal tract, dysplasia which is interpreted as severe or high grade has become recognised as a marker for either increased risk of cancer or for an existing but undiagnosed cancer. Following a diagnosis of high-grade dysplasia, patients may be advised (in the light of other clinical findings, age and state of health) to undergo surgery to either prevent cancer or to remove it in its early and curative stage. Such a decision generally follows confirmation of the diagnosis of dysplasia by two expert pathologists. Radical surgery may now be avoided by the use of local excision techniques. These require visualisation of the lesion by dye spraying methods coupled with high-resolution video-endoscopy. This conservative approach to small and circumscribed foci of gastrointestinal neoplasia (endoscopic mucosal resection) was pioneered in Japan.

The significance of a diagnosis of high-grade dysplasia (in terms of therapeutic options) will be greatly influenced by the feasibility, acceptability and safety of surgical procedures. This in turn will be influenced by the site of the lesion. Given that modern surgery is relatively safe even for deep-seated lesions, that society is becoming increasingly litigious, and that a diagnosis of high-grade dysplasia or carcinoma-in-situ inevitably sets alarm bells ringing, there is a very real possibility of overtreatment and hence of subjecting patients to unnecessary risks. It has been pointed out that estimates of risk for pre-cancer have been derived through studies of small numbers of patients by anatomical pathologists with special expertise. Their advice has subsequently been translated into large-scale practice conducted by non-experts that now proceeds with insufficient review of outcomes (Foucar, 1997).

EARLY CANCER

Once dysplastic cells have traversed the basement membrane and invaded underlying tissues, the neoplasm is regarded as invasive. Is this a stage which should always be labelled as malignant? For example, if an early cancer showing superficial spread is never associated with metastasis, should cancer be diagnosed? There is no consistency here. Colorectal adenomas that include invasive foci which have proceeded no further than the underlying stroma of the lamina propria (i.e. still restricted to the mucous membrane) are termed adenomas with severe dysplasia by many pathologists. Conversely, melanomas showing superficial invasion by small groups of cells that spread horizontally but not deeply are called radial growth phase melanomas, yet have no capacity for metastasis.

How is it that reporting practices vary so much between different lesions associated with similar outcomes? In the case of colorectal adenoma we are considering a lesion that was once not even regarded as precancerous (Spratt & Ackerman, 1962). Aside from the negligible risk of metastasis in early colorectal cancer, this historical background invites a 'benign' attitude in relation to this neoplasm. The opposite approach has been taken in the case of malignant melanoma. Here the starting point was a cancer well known for its aggressiveness. Despite identifying early forms of invasive neoplasia with non-metastatic potential, we seem unable to drop the term cancer in retrospect. Screening for early cancer has now led to cancer epidemics in relation to both prostate cancer and malignant melanoma. But are we necessarily dealing with cancer, or simply stretching morphology beyond acceptable limits for want of rigorous clinical correlation? Screening for early cancer is now providing the pathologist with lesions of uncertain portent and this uncertainty needs to be more widely recognised (Foucar, 1997).

SCREENING FOR CANCER

Cancer screening is the application of a test to an asymptomatic, apparently healthy target population, in order to detect individuals at increased risk of developing of cancer (Reintgen & Clark, 1996). This objective is generally achieved by detecting the neoplasm at a stage when it may be successfully treated (e.g. before it has attained the potential to spread to distant sites). One type of cancer screening involves the demonstration of a risk factor (in the absence of an apparent lesion), such as an inherited or acquired genetic mutation (see Chapter 23), which places an individual at risk of developing cancer in the future. The specific skills of anatomical pathologists may be involved in three distinct areas of screening: (1) in the diagnosis of early neoplastic change (e.g. in cervical cancer screening), (2) in the examination of surgical specimens for the purposes of establishing a diagnosis and the need for further treatment, and (3) in the determination of the natural history of the disease, i.e. the timing of initial onset, the stage when early diagnosis is possible, the stage when usual diagnosis is made on the basis of clinical symptoms, and the various possible outcomes such as recovery, disability or death.

How do we know that these early beginnings will go on to invade normal tissues and spread to distant parts of the body? The most definite proof comes when an early lesion is not removed after detection. In the case of neoplastic polyps (adenomas) of the colon, cancers have subsequently been observed to develop within the polyps of patients who refused intervention (Muto et al., 1975). In the case of the cervix, gynaecologists once elected not to treat the early lesions but to follow them up. The women did not know that anything was wrong, but continued to attend the follow-up clinics. Some women went on to develop invasive cancer of the cervix and some died of the disease (McIndoe et al., 1984). If a cancer is detected a little earlier than usual but not early enough to prevent spread and death, then the test will not influence mortality rates. The resultant increase in survival is apparent only, and is known as 'lead time bias'. Screening tests may be based not on the direct visualisation of cells but on radiology (e.g. breast cancer) or biochemistry (e.g. prostate specific antigen; PSA). In these cases, the anatomical pathologist still provides the definitive tissue diagnosis, for example through the examination of a needle biopsy specimen.

A screening test may fail to detect significant neoplasia. False negative results may occur for a variety of reasons. In the case of cervical cancer screening, the test sample may be inadequate, neoplastic cells may be obscured by other pathology, or the screener may overlook small numbers of neoplastic cells. A test that shows high sensitivity has few false negative results, but 100% sensitivity can never be realised in practice. False positivity (i.e. lack of specificity) is not so problematical in the case of cervical screening, but becomes significant when the test involves the detection of a tumour product such as PSA, or bleeding in the case of colorectal cancer. A raised PSA may be caused by inflammation. Bleeding has numerous causes. Apart from the issues of sensitivity and specificity, a cancer screening test must be acceptable to the target population. It must also, if it is to be effective, be targeted to populations in which the prevalence of the particular form of cancer is high. The incidence of cancer may rise or fall as a result of changes in the environment. A screening test is effective if it reduces the mortality rate independently of a falling disease incidence due to unrelated factors. To demonstrate the effectiveness of a screening test, it must be performed in the context of a clinical trial in which there is a control group that does not receive screening but is in other respects identical to the screened group. Finally, it should be stressed that a screening result can only assign a probability that a disease may already exist or develop in the future and this can never be error-free for an individual. This is because a screening test can never be 100% specific and sensitive.

REFERENCES

Foucar, E. (1997) Do pathologists play dice? Uncertainty and early histopathological diagnosis of common malignancies. *Histopathology,* **31**, 495–502.

McIndoe, W.A., McClean, M.R., Jones, R.W. & Mullins, P.R. (1984) The invasive potential of carcinoma *in situ* of the cervix. *Obstet Gynecol*, **64**, 451–458.

Muto, T., Bussey, H.J.R. & Morson, B.C. (1975) The evolution of cancer of the colon and rectum. *Cancer,* **36**, 2251–2270.

Reintgen, D.S. & Clark, R.A. (1996) *Cancer Screening*. St Louis; Mosby.

Spratt, J.S. & Ackerman, L.V. (1962) Small primary adenocarcinomas of the colon and rectum. *JAMA,* **179**, 337–346.

26

THE MANAGEMENT OF CANCER:
A PATHOLOGIST'S PERSPECTIVE

*The only thing that's been made clear is that your tumour
can be fought, that all is not lost yet*

Alexander Solzhenitsyn *(Cancer Ward)*

Is a diagnosis always correct?

INTEGRATING ROLE FOR THE PATHOLOGIST

This book has described the role of the anatomical pathologist and provided an account of disease that is slanted towards the practice of pathology. Much of the day-to-day work of the anatomical pathologist is devoted to the management of cancer. This reflects the paramount importance of achieving a firm diagnosis of cancer that is based upon the examination of a tissue specimen. The pathological vantage point offers only one particular view of the nature of cancer, this view differing somewhat from the view of the surgeon, the epidemiologist, the cancer researcher or the patient. The surgeon sees cancer as a disease requiring surgical excision, the epidemiologist sees it as a disease responsible for about a quarter of all deaths, the cancer researcher as a disease caused by the disordered function of mutated genes and the patient as a disease that may be associated with a long and painful death. As a heir of Virchow's theories of cellular pathology, the anatomical pathologist will view cancer as a structural and functional disorder of the cell. There is inherent danger in any view that is limited in scope. The anatomical pathologist occupies a somewhat privileged position located at the crossroads of laboratory and clinical medicine, able to rove with relative ease from the world of cells and tissues both 'downwards' to molecules and genes and 'upwards' to individuals, families and populations. Integration may be achieved from such a vantage point.

REMOTE PATHOLOGY AND THE CANCER REPORT

How restricted should the input of the anatomical pathologist be in relation to the management of a patient with cancer? The preceding chapters (21, 22 & 24) have shown how the pathologist is able to extract diagnostic and prognostic information from biopsy or surgical specimens of cancer. The focus has been on the generic knowledge and skills of the pathologist in relation to a defined task. The attitude of the pathologist towards the use of the generated information has not been considered. At one extreme the pathologist could remain in an office and provide accurate microscopic descriptions of each specimen submitted for analysis. These descriptions could be 100% accurate, year in and year out, but is such a 'wise hermit' adequately supporting the needs of the patient?

There are hidden pitfalls associated with what one of my teachers, Basil Morson, described to me as 'postal pathology'—specimens posted in, reports posted out. Firstly, rigid compartmentalisation of anatomical pathology diminishes its relevance to the patient. There is a definite requirement to actively seek and incorporate into one's reasoning all relevant clinical information; this may not necessarily be provided in the request form (see Chapter 4). Secondly, the anatomical pathologist is continually required to re-set diagnostic thresholds; a process which is facilitated by sharing difficult or rare problems with colleagues. Third is the requirement to develop and refine reporting practices as new clinical or pathological understanding comes to light. Fourth is the Hippocratic obligation to teach others by contributing new understanding to the body of literature that underpins the discipline. After all, if previous generations of anatomical pathologists had not established the links between microscopic appearance and behaviour of diseased tissues, the discipline would not exist. The literature has not been fixed as an unchanging truth. Anatomical pathology will continue to evolve as it incorporates new insights from the expanding field of molecular and cellular biology and adjusts itself to the introduction of new therapeutic options.

Although anatomical pathologists may be more retiring than others in the medical profession and therefore inclined towards a 'postal' approach, an additional factor contributing to such a position will be an unreasonably high workload. All anatomical pathologists are capable of reporting large numbers of specimens at a single sitting. However, if this were the only permissible activity, the discipline would gradually ossify into an increasingly meaningless function divorced from clinical reality. Yet in a world of harsh economic rationalisation, it is products (the reports) that generate income. Quality and professional development come second.

DIAGNOSTIC ERRORS

Do anatomical pathologists ever make diagnostic errors? What exactly is meant by an error? In relation to cancer, errors include the diagnosis of a non-malignant disease as cancer, and conversely the failure to appreciate that a lesion is in fact a cancer. The former is the more serious mistake, because it may lead to unnecessary and potentially harmful treatment. The latter is likely to be picked up and result only in a small delay in the treatment of cancer. The cancer may be recognised, but typed incorrectly. This may also lead to inappropriate treatment. Description of the stage or extent of spread may be performed inadequately and this may also disadvantage the patient when the decision to offer or not offer further treatment has to be made in the absence of information that should have been available. A very basic error would be to mistake a mestastatic deposit for a primary cancer. Finally, other variables that could have a bearing on prognosis or treatment may have been neglected by the pathologist. The student or inexperienced pathologist will avoid such errors by asking the following questions:

1. Is the lesion a neoplasm or not?
2. If it is, is it benign or malignant?
3. If it is malignant, is it primary or secondary?
4. What type of neoplasm is it?
5. What additional prognostic information should be provided for this type of neoplasm to allow optimum patient care?

It is most unusual for pathologist to diagnose an innocent lesion as cancer because of the tendency to err on the side of caution. Overdiagnosis of cancer is most likely to occur amongst pathologists working in isolation, for whom diagnostic thresholds have drifted from the norm. A missed diagnosis occurs either through excessive haste or inexperience. Incorrect classification of cancer arises when technical and diagnostic protocols are rudimentary, or through simple ignorance. Limitations on classification are imposed by inadequate material. Awareness of the limits of one's diagnostic abilities, and of when it is appropriate to request an additional sample or seek a further opinion, will render such errors less likely. Complete classification of malignant lymphoma may require samples to be submitted in a fresh state as opposed to a partially fixed state in formaldehyde (see Chapter 3). 'Making do' with inadequate samples will disadvantage a subset of patients with malignant lymphoma. Ignorance of or failure to institute standardised protocols for the dissection and reporting of surgical specimens will account for most of the missing information in reports.

Pathologists have rarely been sued for their errors. This is because reports are taken as representing an opinion and not as a statement of an absolute truth. In addition, it is often very difficult to prove that an individual patient has been disadvantaged by a pathologist's opinion. The obligation to include information that should form part of a standardised report may change this position, particularly when an omission has been shown to disadvantage a patient with cancer.

PATIENT MANAGEMENT

How should the anatomical pathologist best manage his or her time and expertise in order to optimise the care of a patient with cancer? Many pathologists adopt a 'passive–defensive' approach to their work and this is often encouraged and appreciated by their clinical colleagues. By this I mean that pathologists choose to give no advice at all on how the patient should be managed, describing only what they see in the specimen submitted to the laboratory and hoping or assuming that the description will be translated into appropriate action on behalf of the patient. It is easy to see how such an abdication of responsibility could come about. First, in order to give good advice one needs to be fully appraised of the relevant clinical information regarding a patient and at the same time to possess a thorough knowledge of the disease. This is in addition to extracting and providing accurate diagnostic information about a cancer specimen. Possession of all three attributes for every diagnosed case of cancer would require the expenditure of considerable effort. Yet, without this effort the work of the pathologist is reduced to disease labelling and ultimately to losing touch with the meaning that the labels have for the patient.

Although pathologists reach a diagnosis on a specimen at a particular moment in time, all diseases are dynamic and change through time. Cancer is no exception. Although the intervening steps cannot be studied in an individual case, the pathologist derives considerable information from observing change over time. This applies most especially to the earliest (precancerous) phases of tumour development, when the potential for malignant progression may be unclear (see Chapter 25). When there have been sequential biopsies over time the pathologist can (and should) review the entire series and form an opinion on the likely natural history of the lesion. This emphasises the importance of ongoing involvement in patient management (and applies also to non-malignant disease). These efforts must also be made within an increasingly difficult environment, in terms of the growing complexity of medical practice, the pressures of commercialisation and an expanding litigiousness within society.

The pace at which new knowledge is accumulating regarding the molecular basis of disease, including cancer (see Chapter 23), is remarkable. As noted above, the pathologist is in a particularly favourable position for applying these advances to diagnostic practice. The opportunities for pathologists to advance understanding and apply new knowledge to the care of the patient are probably greater now than at any time in history.

THE INTEGRATED TEAM APPROACH

Another issue regarding cancer is the rapidly developing multidisciplinary approach to its management. Once a disease that lent itself almost exclusively to the craft of the surgeon, cancer is increasingly being investigated and managed by other disciplines such as radiology, endoscopy, radiotherapy, clinical oncology, clinical genetics and clinical immunology. Cancer screening and earlier diagnosis have created a 'new' pathology of early cancer (see Chapter 25). Pathology has traditionally been a discipline of pivotal importance in the training programs of surgeons. A declining emphasis on pathology in surgical training over the last decade has been countered by the growing appreciation by other disciplines, notably radiology, radiotherapy and oncology. Pathologists are increasingly honing their expertise towards specific and common forms of cancer, and working with representatives of other disciplines towards integration and standardisation of clinical protocols. Screening, diagnosis and treatment of cancer will be based increasingly on reliable clinical evidence and this will lead to improved outcomes. The reporting of cancer specimens by anatomical pathologists will itself be optimised through standardisation that is evidence-based, and this will ensure that any move towards commercialisation does not lead to a lowering of reporting standards.

— PART V —

MESSENGERS, METABOLISM, MULTISYSTEM AND MECHANICAL DISEASE

GENETIC DISORDERS

Genetics is to biology what the atomic theory is to physical sciences

Victor McKusick

What is the scale of the burden posed by hereditary disorders?

GENETIC DISEASE AND THE PATHOLOGIST

Genetics is the branch of science that studies variation within and between species, and specifically the inherited basis of that variation. The subject is of paramount importance to all medical disciplines. Pathologists may observe and document variation at autopsy and during microscopic examination of tissues that is genetically based. The pathologist may diagnose an inherited disorder at autopsy which was not suspected during the patient's life yet which may be of relevance to the patient's family. The pathologist may also diagnose genetic disorders by the use of special stains to demonstrate abnormal cellular products and cancer, now known to be hereditary in some cases, is diagnosed by the pathologist on a routine basis.

FUNDAMENTALS OF GENETICS AND THE BASIS OF GENETIC DISEASE

It is only within the last few decades that the molecular nature of the gene has been understood and biochemical techniques to study the gene have been made available to scientists. The pioneers of genetic research based their hypotheses on simple observations drawn from nature and were years ahead of their time. Charles Darwin and Alfred Wallace may be placed within this category, but the Moravian monk Gregor Johann Mendel (1822–1884) is rightly regarded as the father of genetics. Even before his time, however the linkage of haemophilia and colour blindness to males had been noted by Otto in Philadelphia and Horner in Germany respectively.

Mendel's principal experimental subject was the common garden pea. He showed how particular characteristics such as tallness were dominant over shortness. The inherited units responsible for these traits were independent. For example, crossing snapdragons with red and white flowers would yield three types of offspring: RR homozygous = red (25%), RW heterozygous = pink (50%) and WW homozygous = white (25%). (Homozygous and heterozygous mean 'same coupling' and 'different coupling' respectively.) The percentages were exact. The independence of the inherited factors R and W was such that seeds from the pink snapdragon (RW) might revert back to red or white flowers, depending on the way the factors were coupled in ensuing generations. Mendel reported his observations and deductions in 1865 in the Czech village of Brno where his monastery garden was located, but his audience failed to comprehend his unusual combination of botany and mathematics, and his pioneering work was ignored for 35 years. After its rediscovery in 1900, his experiments were repeated and found to be reproducible down to the last detail.

It was left to others, notably Theodor Boveri, to demonstrate that the hereditary units resided in the chromosomes. Each species of higher organism was found to have a characteristic number of chromosomes occurring as pairs—one of maternal and the other of paternal origin. The chromosomes were observed to replicate and separate when a cell divided into two (mitosis). While this was true of all somatic cells, germ cells yielded ova or sperm in which the chromosomes occurred singly rather than in pairs. Through meiosis (see Fig. 37) the paired hereditary units (alleles) residing on maternally and paternally derived chromosomes (such as R and W) would revert to their independent status, coupling again with a new partner if an ovum should be fertilised by a sperm.

Thomas Morgan was Professor of Experimental Zoology at Columbia University from 1904 to 1928, and it was during this period that he conducted experiments on the fruitfly *Drosophila melanogaster* that were of far-reaching importance. The advantages of his experimental model were that males and females could be distinguished easily, that the female laid 1000 eggs, that a new generation was produced every twelfth day and that the fly had only four pairs of chromosomes. A large amount of genetic data could therefore be produced readily and interpreted with relative ease.

In the spring of 1910 a mutant male fly appeared from a pedigreed strain with white eyes instead of the usual red. Morgan crossed the white-eyed male with a red-eyed female (exactly as Mendel had done with his peas and snapdragons) and showed that the red-eyed trait could be passed down to male flies but never to female flies. The trait was linked to factors that determined gender (sex-linked). He went on to show that some mutant characteristics (such as yellow wings) were not sex-linked, yet tended to be co-inherited with other factors (such as white eyes). Morgan coined the term gene (meaning race or breed in Greek) for the hereditary units responsible for fruitfly characteristics. He and his associates deduced that genes were arranged in a particular order in the chromosomes like the beads of a necklace. Morgan postulated that during the process of meiosis (Fig. 37), a row of beads from one chromosome was exchanged with the equivalent row of beads from its partner.

This process of crossing-over is now termed recombination, and accounts for much of the variability within species. Further studies have shown that inherited characteristics that are linked must be close together on the chromosome and therefore unlikely to be parted during the process of recombination. The distance between genetic loci on a chromosome is proportional to the recombination frequency expressed as a percentage (known as a centimorgan —named after the discoverer). These insights, for which Morgan received the Nobel prize in physiology and medicine, form the basis of modern gene mapping or positional cloning. Once the position of one gene is known the position of another can be calculated from linkage data. It is interesting to note that this work preceded our understanding of the molecular structure of the gene by five decades.

The main limitation of Morgan's work was the infrequency of spontaneous genetic mutation. His student Herman Muller showed that X-rays could cause mutations, but at a greatly accelerated rate. Muller also hypothesised that spontaneously occurring mutations were caused by the naturally occurring cosmic radiation to which all living organisms are exposed. The resulting mutations provide the variation that supports the process of evolution. The price that is paid for the evolution of a species however is genetic disease, including cancer. Muller received a Nobel prize for his work in 1946 (Bordley & Harvey, 1976).

Archibald Garrod was also years ahead of his time when he proposed the concept of 'inborn errors of metabolism' in 1909. He suggested (based on his work on the disorder alkaptonuria) that mutated genes gave rise to defective enzymes, and proposed that inborn errors of metabolism were inherited as Mendelian recessive traits (requiring the inheritance of two inactive genes). He was right, but thirty years were to pass before enzymes were shown to be proteins, and a further two decades were to elapse before the genetic coding mechanism for protein synthesis was discovered. Now, many hundreds of such inborn errors of metabolism are known, each being caused by recessive genes as predicted by Garrod.

DNA AND MUTATIONS

Turning to the molecular structure of the gene, the nucleus of each cell of the human body contains 23 pairs of chromosomes, a maternal and a paternal chromosome contributing to

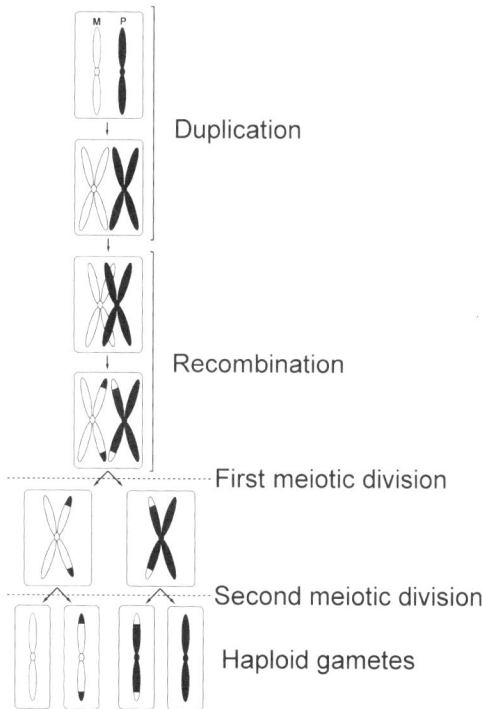

Figure 37 Steps in meiotic cell division

each pair. Chromosomes are made up of a complex chemical called deoxyribose nucleic acid or DNA. DNA is in turn made up of two long chains of units called bases entwined together as the now famous double helix described initially by Watson and Crick (1953) (Fig. 38). There are only four bases: adenine (A), thymine (T), guanine (G) and cytosine (C). The bases of one chain are paired with the bases of the other, A to T and G to C. Within each chromosome are millions of such base pairs, perhaps around 100 million depending on the size of the chromosome. Certain sequences of base pairs serve as templates for the synthesis of proteins. The genetic instruction is carried by an intermediary messenger, called mRNA, from the DNA in the nucleus to the ribosomal RNA within the rough endoplasmic reticulum of surrounding cytoplasm, which is the site of protein synthesis. Genes, the working units within chromosomes, are the special sequences of codons in DNA that code for proteins. Most of the remaining chromosomal material (the great majority) has no known function and can be likened to junk mail.

Whereas DNA is made of only four bases, proteins are built of 20 amino acids. The DNA code works through a series of three bases serving as a template for one amino acid. Three such adjacent bases are known as a codon. Mutations frequently involve a single base within a codon. For example, one base may be substituted by an inappropriate base, such as a C instead of a T. This tiny change may then send out the wrong message (a missense mutation). Typically, the altered codon may code for a different amino acid, which may in turn

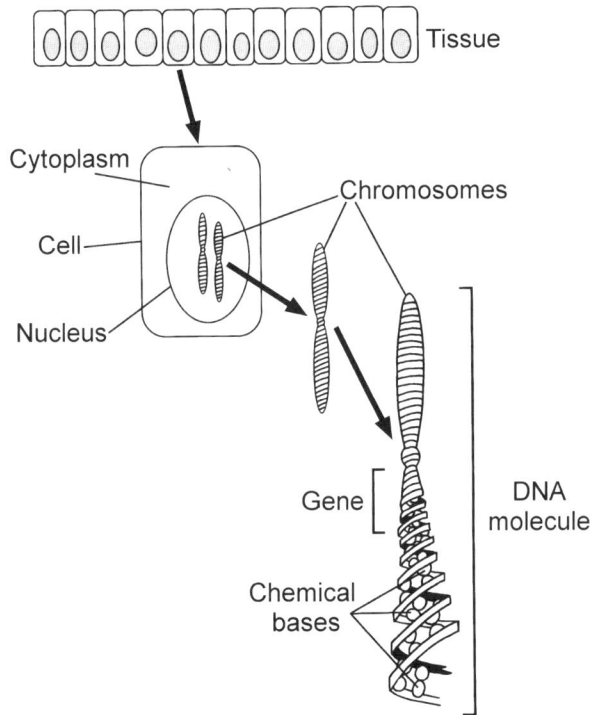

Figure 38 Unraveling chromosomal coils to reveal the double stranded helical structure of DNA

alter the structure and function of the protein. Alternatively, the mutation could order the synthesis of the protein to stop prematurely (by becoming a specific stop signal, or as a nonsense mutation), resulting in the production of a 'truncated protein'. A nucleotide may be added or deleted resulting in a frameshift mutation (disrupting downstream coding completely and again causing protein truncation). It is also possible that the mutation could have no significant consequences (silent mutation). Given that each chromosome has many millions of bases, an error in only one (called a point mutation) will be extremely difficult to find. It is like being asked to find a single misprinted letter in a dictionary. The technology for detecting such a small error certainly exists, but the task is onerous and there are many pitfalls. Larger mutations, for example the deletion of a long run of bases, may be equally difficult to detect.

Until comparatively recently clinical genetics has been regarded as a 'Cinderella' specialty, focusing on rare, unpleasant, incurable and socially disturbing diseases. Not only has the subject been given little attention by the medical profession, but the vociferous public health sector has ensured that environmental agents have been seen as the main culprits in the causation of disease. Yet an individual's genetic constitution may not only include major single gene defects but may also modify disease risks in a multitude of ways. These will include the efficacy of the immune response, the metabolic handling of dietary factors and other environmental agents and the ability to repair damaged DNA. Virtually all disease has a genetic as well as an environmental basis.

ANATOMICAL PATHOLOGISTS AND GENETIC DISEASE

Autosomal dominant conditions are passed from parent to child with each child having a 50% chance of inheriting the altered gene. Such conditions are therefore easy to recognise, particularly because they are often associated with obvious physical and/or mental changes. Pathologists have generally contributed to the recognition of autosomal dominant conditions associated with internal abnormalities such as neoplasia. This has come about either through autopsy practice, in which connections have been made between multiple and apparently unrelated lesions, and/or through the pathologist's traditional interest in cancer.

Friedrich von Recklinghausen (1833–1910), a successor of Virchow, published his classic account of neurofibromatosis type I in 1882 on the basis of autopsy findings in a woman aged 55 and a man aged 47 years. Aldred Warthin served as Professor of Pathology at the University of Michigan Medical Center from 1903 until his death in 1931. He was alerted to the existence of hereditary internal malignancy when his glum seamstress informed him that she was doomed to die of cancer at an early age (which she did). Her large family (with numerous living descendants) is now known to be affected with the condition hereditary non-polyposis colorectal cancer (HNPCC). Warthin (1913) emphasised the importance of linking a firm tissue diagnosis with family history, and conducted his research on material that was population based. His message relating to the misleading inaccuracy of death certification in clinical research remains valid today (Start et al., 1997).

Although the association of thyroid carcinoma with pheochromocytoma (neoplasm of the adrenal medulla secreting adrenaline and noradrenaline) had been documented earlier in several case reports, Williams (1965) showed that the thyroid cancers were medullary carcinomas composed of endocrine cells secreting the hormone calcitonin (which blocks the release of calcium from bone), that the pheochromocytomas often involved both adrenals within a single individual, that the tumours ran in families and that the underlying defect was likely to be a genetic mutation expressed within the cells of the neuroendocrine system. The additional feature of nerve tumours of the oral mucosa and gastrointestinal tract was added subsequently to the autosomal dominant syndrome now known as multiple endocrine neoplasia type IIB (Williams & Pollock, 1966).

The names of several neuropathologists are linked to a cluster of degenerative conditions of the central nervous system which were appreciated either at the time or subsequently to have a genetic component. These include Friedrich (1825–1882), Jakob (1884–1931), Creutzfeldt (1885–1964) and Alzheimer (1864–1915).

The recognition of autosomal recessive 'inborn errors of metabolism' lagged behind the insightful perceptions of Garrod and the documentation of the autosomal dominant conditions. The names of two pathologists, Niemann (1880–1921) and Pick (1868–1944), are associated with a group of conditions characterised by the abnormal accumulation of lipids (sphingomyelin and cholesterol) in the lysosomes of macrophages of the spleen and other organs. The cells may be identified at the light microscope level by applying fat stains to frozen sections, and at the level of the electron microscope by the presence of 'zebra-bodies' within the lysosomes. Some of the glycogen storage diseases are named after anatomical pathologists including von Gierke's (1877–1945) type I (hepatic type due to glucose-6-phosphatase deficiency) and Pompe's (1901–1944) type II (generalised distribution including muscle and due to lysosomal glucosidase deficiency).

The deaths of so many of the aforementioned pathologists around 1945 was not a coincidence. Despite having served in the German army in World War I, Ludwig Pick was imprisoned in the notorious Theresienstadt concentration camp where he died at the age of 76 years. Johannes Pompe was a Dutch patriot who was executed by the Nazis at the age of 44 years after he blew up a strategic railway line. Edgar von Gierke died of natural causes but worked in his retirement with a terminal illness at the Karlsruhe General Hospital after his successor had been drafted into the crumbling German army. Hans-Gerhard Creutzfeldt allowed his clinic to be used as a refuge by Nazi victims but his wife was imprisoned by the Nazis (Beighton & Beighton, 1986).

We have referred to the contribution by pathologists to the recognition of inherited disorders. At the diagnostic front, anatomical pathology, like so many other clinical disciplines, must work closely with both classical genetics and the new molecular genetics. For genetic disorders that were formerly diagnosed on the basis of morphological change, including the histochemical demonstration of abnormal metabolic products, the gold standard will increasingly shift towards the detection of specific mutations. Nevertheless, in cases where the metabolic product is easily picked up by the pathologist or is toxic, such as the iron that accumulates in the liver of subjects with haemochromatosis (perhaps the most common genetic disorder), the anatomical pathologist will continue to play a key role.

The diagnosis of tumours is continuously being refined by the addition of molecular genetic and cytogenetic studies. The demonstration of gene rearrangements is indicative of clonality and helps to confirm the fact of neoplasia. This has proved useful in the case of the recognition and typing of malignant lymphoma and can be achieved by the use of relatively simple approaches employing the polymerase chain reaction (PCR) (see page 158). A number of cancers, particularly leukaemias, tumours of childhood and connective tissue tumours (sarcomas), are characterised by specific rearrangements at the chromosomal level (such as translocations) which can be demonstrated by classical karyotyping or by the use of fluorescent in situ hybridisation (FISH). These techniques require dividing cells, and tumour samples must be sent to the laboratory fresh and not in the usual formalin solution. Other genetic changes may serve as prognostic markers or indicate the likely responses to treatment.

Many cancers contain multiple extra chromosomes (aneuploidy), but a subset of certain commonly occurring cancers shows DNA microsatellite instability (MSI) with a near normal chromosomal distribution (diploidy). Not only may these two broad groups of cancers (aneuploid versus MSI) differ in tumour prognosis and behaviour, but a proportion of the latter will be caused by an inherited germline mutation within a DNA mismatch repair gene (this condition is called HNPCC; see page 159). In the case of HNPCC as well as in other forms of inherited cancer, the anatomical pathologist is able to recognise subtle but discriminatory differences at the light microscopic level. Large bowel cancer in HNPCC tends to be right sided (caecum, ascending or transverse colon), poorly differentiated or mucinous, well circumscribed and peppered with intra-epithelial lymphocytes. Breast cancers caused by *BRCA1* mutations are also likely to be undifferentiated, circumscribed, associated with lymphocytes and have a high mitotic rate (so-called medullary carcinomas). Inherited cancers may also include highly specific types, such as medullary carcinoma of the thyroid. The anatomical pathologist will often be the first to suspect a diagnosis of hereditary cancer (Jass, 1997).

GENOMIC IMPRINTING

Genes of maternal and paternal origin should, according to the laws of Mendel, display identical activity. It is now apparent that some genes may be expressed differently according to the parent of origin. The silencing of a gene derived from a particular parent is called genomic imprinting. Imprinting occurs before fertilisation and is transmitted in a stable manner in the somatic cells of an individual. However, passage of a paternally imprinted gene into a female offspring, for example, will result in reversal of imprinting during oogenesis. Imprinting occurs by methylation of DNA (see page 161), and is reversed by demethylation.

Genomic imprinting may be suspected on clinical grounds when an inherited disease occurs in both males and females but is transmitted only by parents of a particular gender. Genomic imprinting may also be suspected when a disease arises *do novo* and is associated with parental disomy (in which an individual has two identical chromosomes derived from the same parent). Interestingly, both scenarios have been observed in the case of the Beckwith-Wiedemann syndrome, an inherited disorder associated with organomegaly, hemihypertrophy, gigantism and a propensity to tumours of childhood, notably nephroblastoma or Wilms' tumour. Underlying this syndrome is the phenomenon of imprinting of the insulin-like growth factor 2 (*IGF2*) gene in female germ cells. A paternal disomy involving the locus 11p15.5 leads to a double dose of *IGF2*. This in turn accounts for the organ enlargement. Conversely, mutations or cytogenetic abnormalities involving the 11p15.5 locus are thought to block the process of imprinting in the female germline. Females and their offspring may therefore possess two functioning copies of *IGF2* and so express a double dose of the growth factor (Tycko, 1997).

REFERENCES

Beighton, P. & Beighton, G. (1986) *The Man Behind the Syndrome*. Berlin: Springer.

Bordley, J. III. & Harvey, A.M. (1976) *Two Centuries of American Medicine*. Philadelphia: Saunders.

Garrod, A.(1909) *Inborn Errors of Metabolism*. London: Oxford Medical Publications.

Jass, J.R. (1997) Origins of familial cancer: histopathological perspectives. *J Clin Pathol*, **50**, 892–895.

Start, R.D., Bury, J.P., Strachan, A.G., Cross, S.S. & Underwood, J.C.E. (1997) Evaluating the reliability of causes of death in published clinical research. *BMJ*, **314**, 271.

Tycko, B. (1997) Genomic imprinting in human pathology. In *Progress in Pathology*, volume 3, edited by N. Kirkham & N.R. Lemoine, pp. 189–210. Edinburgh: Churchill Livingstone.

Warthin, A.S. (1913) Heredity with reference to carcinoma as shown by the study of the cases examined in the pathological laboratory of the University of Michigan, 1895–1913. *Arch Int Med*, **12**, 546–555.

Watson, J.D. & Crick, F.H.C. (1953) Molecular structure of nucleic acids. A structure for deoxyribose nucleic acid. *Nature,* **171**, 737–738.

Williams, E.D. (1965) A review of 17 cases of carcinoma of the thyroid and phaeochromocytoma. *J Clin Pathol,* **18**, 288–292.

Williams, E.D. & Pollock, D.J. (1966) Multiple mucosal neuromata with endocrine tumours: a syndrome allied to von Recklinghansen's disease. *J Pathol Bacteriol,* **90**, 71–80.

28

DEVELOPMENTAL DISORDERS

When people see some things as beautiful, other things seem ugly

Tao Te Ching

To what extent is a neoplasm a disorder of development?

INTRODUCTION

The pathology of development encompasses processes related to extra-embryonic tissues (placenta), formation of the embryo (embryogenesis), growth of the fetus, birth and adaptation to life outside the uterus (Wigglesworth, 1992). In this brief overview the focus will be on problems presenting at or after birth. The principal categories are congenital malformations and tumours of a developmental nature. Distinction must be made between hereditary disorders which could recur in subsequent pregnancies, and those with a poly-genic or environmental aetiology for which the risk of recurrence is not increased significantly.

CONGENITAL MALFORMATIONS

Congenital malformations have been known to humankind since the dawn of time. Serious malformations are due to a localised error of structural development occurring in the eight weeks following conception. Milder defects (included in Table 10) develop later. One malfor-mation may lead to another and be caused by genetic factors, by environmental factors or by a combination of the two. The genetic causes are classified into chromosomal and single gene disorders. A chromosomal disorder implies an abnormality that can be visualised by the technique of preparing a chromosome spread from a dividing cell and examining the stained chromosomes under a microscope (karyotyping). Abnormalities may include an extra chro-mosome (e.g. trisomy 21 causing Down's syndrome), an absent chromosome (e.g. XO causing Turner's syndrome), deletion of part of a chromosome, inversion of part of a chromosome or a translocation of one part of a chromosome to another. Chromosomal disorders usually arise during gametogenesis and are generally not transmitted since affected individuals either die at birth or are sterile.

Single gene disorders may be autosomal-dominant, autosomal-recessive or sex-linked. Most of the genetic abnormalities that are lethal at or soon after birth are autosomal recessive, for example infantile polycystic kidney disease. The majority of common malformations, however, are considered to be polygenic (caused by the interactions of multiple genes), though environmental factors such as deficiency of the vitamin folic acid are also likely to be implicated. The risks to subsequent pregnancies must be established so that parents can be offered genetic counselling.

The environmental causes of malformation include drugs, chemicals and infections. Agents responsible for congenital malformations are called teratogens and include drugs used in cancer therapy (folate antagonists and alkylating agents), androgenic steroids, alcohol and thalidomide. Rubella virus is most teratogenic at 8-10 weeks, when it causes growth retardation, microphthalmia (abnormal eye development) and heart defects. Persistence of the virus will lead to additional abnormalities such as deafness. Other infective agents that may cause structural defects are *Treponema pallidum* (the cause of syphilis), *Toxoplasma*, Cytomegalovirus and Herpesvirus.

DEVELOPMENTAL TUMOURS

Developmental tumours are a rare cause of death in the perinatal period but some may be lethal in childhood. The three main types of developmental tumour are hamartomas, teratomas and the family of malignant tumours of childhood or 'blastomas' (see page 146). A hamartoma is a tumour-like mass formed of an excess of disorganised tissues normally found

Table 10 Developmental defects

Type	Definition	Examples
Ectopia (or heterotopia)	Occurrence of tissue or organ outside its normal site	Columnar epithelium in upper oesophagus. Gastric epithelium in Meckel's diverticulum
Atresia	Failure to form a lumen	Regions of gut including oesophagus and small intestine
Agenesis	Total failure in organ or tissue development	Examples of organ agenesis include cerebellum and kidney
Aplasia	Absence of organ with persistence of embryonic remnant	Pulmonary aplasia
Hypoplasia	Incomplete development leading to a reduction in size of an organ or structure	Small eyes (microphthalmia) Small jaw (micrognathia) Small head (microcephaly)
Dysraphia	Failure of fusion of opposite structures (right and left) in the midline	Spina bifida

at the site of origin of the mass. The concept of developmental tumours raises the question of the relationship between maldevelopment and neoplasia. Recent observations such as the following are beginning to blur distinctions that were once held rigidly:

- Many inherited syndromes due to single gene defects produce malformations in some organs and neoplasms in others.
- Mutations involving cancer genes are being described with increasing frequency in focal lesions described as hamartomatous, hyperplastic, metaplastic or cystic.
- Genes implicated in the control of embryological development have been shown to serve as tumour suppressor genes (e.g. *cdx2* and *ptc*) (Hahn et al., 1996; Wicking et al., 1998).
- A number of lesions have always fallen between the categories of simple hamartomas and bona fide neoplasms (e.g. haemangiomas, pigmented nevi of the skin and neurofibromas).

Developmental disorders are the province of the paediatric pathologist working in close association with cytogenetic services. Nevertheless, the more minor developmental lesions may be diagnosed in adult life. Many of these present as 'tumours'. Consequently, there is likely to be a major revision of the premises upon which tumours are classified in the near future. The concept of neoplasia will need to be broadened to include some that rarely if ever progress to cancer, others that have a low risk and a group with a higher risk of progression. The principal characteristic unifying neoplasia will be a localised disorder of growth caused by one or more genetic mutations.

REFERENCES

Hahn, H., Wicking, C., Zephiropoulos, P.G., Gailani, M.R., Shanley, S., Chidambaram, A., Vorechovski, I., Holmberg, E., Unden, A.B. & Gillies, S., et al. (1996) Mutations of the human homolog of *Drosophila* patched in the nevoid basal cell carcinoma syndrome. *Cell,* **85**, 841–851.

Wicking, C., Simms, L.A., Evans, T., Walsh, M., Chawengsaksophak, K., Beck, F., Chenevix-Trench, G., Young, J., Jass, J.R., Leggett, B. & Wainwright, B. (1998) *CDX2*, a human homologue of caudal, is mutated in both alleles in a replication error positive colorectal cancer. *Oncogene,* **17**, 657–659.

Wigglesworth, J.S. (1992) Principles of developmental pathology. In *Oxford Textbook of Pathology*, volume 1, edited by J.O'D. McGee, P.G. Isaacson & N.A. Wright, pp. 781–792. Oxford: Oxford University Press.

Further reading

Keeling, J.W (ed) (1993) *Fetal and Neonatal Pathology* (2nd edn). London: Springer-Verlag.

29

THE ENDOCRINE SYSTEM:
SOLID AND DIFFUSE

*I do hope it'll make me grow large again, for really
I'm quite tired of being such a tiny little thing*

Alice

Why are endocrine disorders difficult to diagnose?

THE EXPANDING ENDOCRINE CONCEPT

Endocrine disorders are a large topic that will be considered here generically and mainly in relation to the structural changes within endocrine glands. The concept of chemical messengers has expanded considerably since the early view of the endocrine gland as an organ that manufactures and secretes hormones into the bloodstream in order to regulate metabolic activities in distant sites. Chemical messengers may operate over much shorter distances, as occurs in the case of the diffuse endocrine system composed of single scattered cells found in such organs as the gut, lung, testis, ovary and prostate. The local effect of secreted hormones is sometimes described as paracrine. A secretion may even act on the cell of origin (autocrine effect). When the cells of the diffuse endocrine system are imagined as a mass, their total volume will be greater than that of the solid endocrine organs.

The locally acting hormones produced by the diffuse endocrine system have exact counterparts within the nervous system and the close working relationship of the nervous and endocrine systems, is now well recognised. However, these are not the only systems containing cells that influence other cells by means of chemical mediators. The cells of the immune system (see Chapter 14) and even platelets (see Chapter 17) fall into this category. In retrospect, the originators of the term 'hormone', Bayliss and Starling, may have had an inkling of the universal nature of the chemical messenger. The word comes from a Greek word which may be translated as 'I arouse to activity', aptly describing all those chemicals that pass from one cell to another for the purposes of activating and orchestrating the biological processes that underlie life (Bayliss, 1924).

The idea that one organ may influence another has been known since antiquity. Eunuchs were favoured as servants and as supervisors of harems in ancient cultures of the Far East, Middle East as well as by the Romans. Up until the eighteenth century castrati were favoured as opera singers. The widespread physiological and psychological effects could scarcely have gone unnoticed. The association of thyroid enlargement with stunted growth and mental impairment was first noted by Felix Platter in Switzerland in 1602 (Bordley & Harvey, 1976).

ENDOCRINE DYSFUNCTION

Diseases attributable to endocrine cell function fall into two main classes:

1.   Overproduction of hormone

This may apply to both the solid and the diffuse endocrine systems. A common cause in both is the formation of a neoplasm (benign or malignant) in which hormone secretion becomes autonomous or removed from normal physiological control. Alternatively an endocrine gland such as the adrenal (cortex) or thyroid may be driven by a chemical messenger that serves to stimulate overgrowth and overactivity. In the case of the adrenal cortex this may be due to the uncontrolled synthesis of ACTH by a pituitary adenoma, whereas the thyroid gland in Graves' disease is driven by an auto-antibody which binds to the TSH receptor.

2.   Underproduction of hormone

This may result from a number of mechanisms which are tabulated for the pituitary, thyroid and adrenal glands (Table 11). Additionally, the underlying causes of endocrine failure of the pituitary, adrenal and thyroid are seen to be very different. In fact, disseminated intravascular coagulation (page 115) accounts for the adrenal destruction in meningococcal septicemia and may also underlie, in part, pituitary infarction. Hyperplasia of the pituitary during pregnancy may cause vascular compression, thereby rendering the gland more susceptible to the effects of shock (Sheehan's syndrome). Its small size and location within the bony confines of the sella may account for the pituitary's predisposition to destruction by local neoplastic processes. The presence of steroids in high concentration within the adrenal cortex may lead to local immunosuppression and therefore to extensive involvement by tuberculosis or fungal infection (histoplasmosis, cryptococcosis or blastomycosis).

Both overproduction and underproduction of hormones have serious and life-threatening metabolic consequences. However, changes often occur slowly and insidiously so that neither the patient nor their family is aware of the problem. A doctor or a friend who has not seen the affected subject for some time may be the first to notice, for example, the changes associated with thyroid failure (coarse skin, croaky voice, thinning hair, slowing up and intellectual impairment), or the gradual overgrowth of bone and soft tissue in acromegaly caused by a growth hormone secreting tumour of the pituitary. Alternatively, the symptoms may be abrupt and catastrophic, such as metabolic collapse and coma in diabetes mellitus and adrenal failure, soaring blood pressure caused by the adrenaline and noradrenaline released by a neoplasm of the adrenal medulla (phaeochromocytoma), or acute heart failure in the acromegalic. However, such acute episodes will usually have been preceded by many months or years of metabolic dysfunction.

Table 11 Causes of endocrine failure of pituitary gland, adrenals and thyroid

Mechanism	Pituitary	Adrenal	Thyroid
(1) Infection/inflammation acute	Rare	Meningococcus Other cocci (rare)	–
chronic	Sarcoidosis	Tuberculosis Cryptococcosis Other fungal	De Quervain's granulomatous thyroiditis (? viral)*
(2) Vascular	Infarction (Sheehan's syndrome)	–	–
(3) Neoplastic primary	Chromophobe adenoma Craniopharyngioma Others (rare)	–	–
metastatic	Various	Rare cause	–
(4) Genetic	–	Congenital metabolic defects (adrenogenital syndromes)	Congenital metabolic defects
(5) Developmental	–	–	Congenital absence
(6) Endocrine	–	Pituitary failure (ACTH)	Hypothalamic failure (TRH) Pituitary failure (TSH)
(7) Nutritional	–	–	Iodine deficiency
(8) Autoimmune	–	Addison's disease (70%)	Hashimoto's disease**
(9) Iatrogenic	Surgery Radiation	Surgery	Surgery Drugs Radiation
(10) Mechanical	Empty sella syndrome	–	–
(11) Idiopathic	–	–	End stage atrophy Riedel's thyroiditis

* Hypothyroidism only when there is severe destruction of thyroid parenchyma (rare). Hyperthyroidism may also occur.

** May also be associated with hyperthyroidism in the early stages.

ENDOCRINE NEOPLASMS

The endocrine disorders that are of most relevance to the anatomical pathologist are the neoplasms. As noted above, these may be derived from cells of both the solid and the diffuse endocrine systems. Neoplasms may synthesise hormones in an excessive and uncontrolled manner, but many endocrine neoplasms are non-functioning. Although a functioning cell may be construed as being closer to normal, some functioning endocrine tumours are malignant, particularly those of the diffuse endocrine system of the gut. Conversely, many non-functioning endocrine neoplasms are benign. The principal distinguishing features of benign and malignant neoplasms are described in Chapter 22, but are often of limited value in relation to endocrine neoplasms.

Perhaps the main role of the anatomical pathologist in the case of functioning neoplasms is in the management of parathyroid disease. Overproduction of parathyroid hormone results in an elevated serum calcium. Such overproduction may be due to a solitary adenoma (the usual cause of primary hyperparathyroidism) or to overgrowth of all four parathyroids. The latter usually occurs in subjects with renal failure as a compensation to a low serum calcium (secondary hyperparathyroidism). This may keep the serum calcium within the normal range, but at the expense of the bones of the body which are stripped of calcium stores. Eventually one or more of the glands may become neoplastic and function autonomously, producing excessive parathyroid hormone, and the serum calcium will increase (tertiary hyperparathroidism). In the case of a parathyroid adenoma the remaining three glands will undergo atrophy and fatty replacement. The surgeon will remove the gland with the adenoma and inspect and biopsy the other three. The pathologist examines frozen sections during the surgical procedure to confirm the diagnosis. More extensive surgery will be required if all four glands are overactive.

Neoplasms of the diffuse endocrine system

Neoplasms of the diffuse endocrine system often cause confusion and slip through the curricular net. The endocrine system has been divided into 'endocrine' and 'neuroendocrine'. Certain common features have been ascribed to neuroendocrine cells: embryological derivation from the neural crest, synthesis of peptide hormones (composed of amino acids), sharing of a particular peptide hormone with cells of the nervous system, diffuse location (often), a granular cytoplasm that may be stained with silver techniques (argyrophil and sometimes argentaffin), cytoplasmic vesicles that are electron dense at the electron microscopic level ('neurosecretory' granules) and the biochemical property of Amine Precursor Uptake and Decarboxylation (APUD). The tumours of this system were described as apudomas (Polak & Bloom, 1985). When this theory was in its heyday, APUD cells were thought to include all the endocrine cells of the gut, pancreas, lung, ovary, testis, prostate and thyroid (calcitonin producing C-cells), cells of the adrenal medulla, cells of the anterior pituitary, cells of the carotid body and the melanocytes of the skin. Whilst some of these cells may be derived from the neural crest (cells of the adrenal medulla and melanocytes), others such as those of the gut are of endodermal origin and the designation neuroendocrine is therefore inappropriate. Strictly speaking, the APUD and neuroendocrine concepts are no longer valid in the original global sense, though the sharing of specialised features (gene expression) by endocrine and neural cells cannot be denied. Additionally a number of autosomal dominant syndromes (such as MEN IIB) are characterised by the development of both endocrine and neural tumours (see Chapter 27).

Another potential source of confusion is the term 'carcinoid' tumour. This has been applied in a narrow sense to the yellow-coloured, slow-growing endocrine tumours of the midgut (ileum and appendix) which secrete the amine 5-hydroxytryptamine (5-HT). The carcinoid syndrome arises when these tumours (usually of the ileum, rarely of the appendix) metastasise to the liver, and non-metabolised 5-HT spreads via the hepatic veins to the heart and the rest of the body. This results in damage and fibrosis of the heart valves, intestinal hypermotility and flushing. The term carcinoid (coined by Oberndorder in 1907) implied that the tumours looked like epithelial neoplasms (carcinomas) at the light microscopic but behaved in a benign fashion. The carcinoid 'look' refers to cells with a cytoplasm containing small eosinophilic granules and nuclei that are round, uniform, stippled and mitotically inactive. The cells do not typically form glands but rather islands, nests or ribbons. In other words these neoplasms look nothing like carcinomas! Moreover, endocrine tumours with the carcinoid look that arise in the small intestine and pancreas are often malignant. Carcinoid or endocrine tumours of the gut, pancreas, lung and other sites are classified as malignant neoplasms, though some, such as the small, incidentally discovered carcinoids of the appendix and rectum, rarely behave in malignant fashion.

Endocrine neoplasms of the gut and pancreas may secrete hormones that produce specific syndromes (Table 12). The neoplasms are often named after the hormone, for example insulinoma and glucagonoma of the pancreas. Endocrine neoplasms may also secrete hormones not normally associated with the tissue of origin (such as gastrinoma of the pancreas). They may also secrete two or more hormones. The presence of different hormones can be demonstrated by means of immunohistochemistry.

Carcinoid tumours of the appendix are very common, but endocrine tumours and particularly those that behave in a malignant fashion are otherwise relatively uncommon. This applies to both the solid and the diffuse endocrine systems.

SYSTEMIC EFFECTS OF DISEASE

Localised diseases often produce generalised or systemic effects. Endocrine disorders and endocrine neoplasms are an obvious example of this phenomenon. Some non-endocrine cancers may produce hormones inappropriately, and the associated metabolic changes (e.g. due to the ectopic production of ACTH, PTH or ADH) may be the first sign of cancer. 'Paraneoplastic' syndromes may arise through other mechanisms such as autoimmune reactions directed towards tumour antigens. Non-specific symptoms including pyrexia, malaise and weight loss are common in both inflammatory and neoplastic conditions. Circulating cytokines such as TNF-α and IL-1 contribute to these systemic effects, but further research is required to elucidate the underlying mechanisms involved. Discovering an underlying cause for vague and generalised symptoms is always a difficult diagnostic challenge.

REFERENCES

Bayliss, W.M. (1924) *Principles of General Physiology*. London: Longmans, Green and Co.
Bordley, J. III. & Harvey, A.M. (1976) *Two Centuries of American Medicine 1777–1976*. Philadelphia: Saunders.
Polak, J.M. & Bloom, S.R. (1985) *Endocrine Tumours. The Pathobiology of Regulatory Peptide-producing Tumours*. Edinburgh: Churchill Livingstone.

Table 12 Neuroendocrine tumours and their syndromes

Tumour	Hormone or amine	Location	Syndrome
Carcinoid	5-hydroxytryptamine (and other amines and vasoactive peptides)	Midgut (ileum, appendix)	Carcinoid syndrome following metastasis to liver: Diarrhoea, flushing, bronchospasm, lesions of the heart valves
Gastrinoma*	Gastrin	Pancreas, duodenum	Zollinger-Ellison syndrome: Multiple peptic ulcers
Insulinoma	Insulin	Pancreas (β cells)	Hypoglycemia
Glucagonoma*	Glucagon	Pancreas (α cells)	Diabetes mellitus, weight loss, red tongue, depression
VIPoma*	Vasoactive intestinal peptide	Pancreas	Verner-Morrison syndrome: Weight loss, watery diarrhoea, hypokalemia
Somatostatinoma*	Somatostatin	Pancreas, duodenum steatorrhoea	Diabetes, hypochlorhydria**

* Tumours likely to be malignant in the absence of demonstrable metastases
** Reduced secretion of gastric acid

30

TUMOUR IMMUNITY,
GRAFT VERSUS HOST DISEASE
AND AUTOIMMUNE DISEASE

You are good when you are at one with yourself

Kahlil Gibran

What is the relationship between hypersensitivity and autoimmune disease?

INTRODUCTION

There are three situations in which host tissue may be a target for immune attack. The autoimmune diseases represent the most obvious example. Secondly, the introduction of bone marrow transplantation provides contaminating T lymphocytes with the unwanted opportunity to mount an attack upon host tissues (graft versus host disease). We will begin, however, with the topic of tumour immunity (the tumour as self) even though it is still unclear how successful the immune system is in either preventing cancer or modifying its behaviour.

TUMOUR IMMUNITY

Anatomical pathologists have long observed and described the presence of inflammatory cells, notably lymphocytes, macrophages and eosinophils, in and around cancers. This finding has been correlated with tumour regression, for example in malignant melanoma, and with improved prognosis. Following Burnet's pioneering work on immune tolerance (page 85), the immune system came to be regarded not only as a defence against infection but also as a system of immunosurveillance that would detect and eliminate cancer cells before they had a chance to proliferate into a recognisable lesion. This view has been given fresh impetus with the introduction of 'psychoimmunobiology'. Even if, as appears likely, the function of the immune system can be shown to be influenced by mental state, there is surprisingly little evidence that immune mechanisms can inhibit early cancer development. Immunity is deliberately suppressed in patients who have received organ transplants. Such patients are at increased risk of certain cancers (e.g. squamous cell carcinoma of skin and lymphoma), but are not at increased risk of developing any of the common and life-threatening forms of cancer. Ultraviolet radiation is also thought to depress skin immunity locally and perhaps add to skin cancer risk by this mechanism. Cancer is an age-related disease and does not threaten breeding efficiency. Therefore there is no evolutionary pressure to acquire a system of cancer immunosurveillance.

The cell membrane of cancer cells express a variety of new antigens: viral antigens, developmental gene products that have been switched back on inappropriately (e.g. alpha fetoprotein) and post-translational changes to the carbohydrate component of cell membrane receptors. Even mutated genetic material may be transported to the cell membrane by MHC class II molecules (see page 88). Although the immune system detects and responds to various cancer antigens, the outcome is not activation of cytotoxic T cells and natural killer cells, but immune tolerance. In the case of infection, antigen presenting cells (see page 89) pick up danger signals in the form of inflammatory cytokines such as GM-CSF (granulocyte-monocyte colony stimulating factor) and TNF-α (tumour necrosis factor-α), and are thereby prompted to activate T cells. On the other hand, tumour antigens that are not co-expressed with such inflammatory mediators are processed by dendritic cells and presented to T cells, but in a form that induces immune tolerance rather than activation.

The possibility of augmenting the immune response came to light as early as 1893, when William Coley observed regression of cancer by the deliberate introduction of infection (Scott & Sebon, 1997). Today superficial bladder cancer is treated by means of immune stimulation with BCG, an attenuated form of *Mycobacterium tuberculosis*. Injections of monoclonal antibodies directed towards cancer cells have led to the improved survival of patients with advanced bowel cancer and melanoma. However, the future lies with the development of vaccines engineered around specific tumour antigens that will activate T cells in the presence of modern molecular adjuvants.

GRAFT VERSUS HOST DISEASE

Graft versus host disease is an unwanted side effect of bone marrow transplantation that results in immune mediated damage. This occurs in an acute form presenting with fever, anaemia, weight loss, skin rashes and diarrhoea. Tissue changes are observed in the skin, gut and liver. Rectal biopsy is a convenient way of confirming the diagnosis, and shows apoptosis affecting the crypt base cells and 'disappearing' crypts. These changes are mediated by cytokines such as TNF-α (tumour necrosis factor-α). A chronic form of the disease resembles the multi-organ autoimmune disease scleroderma in which there is abnormal collagen deposition within connective tissues resulting in tightening and contraction.

AUTOIMMUNE DISEASE

The term autoimmune disease refers to a miscellaneous group of disorders in which hypersensitivity is directed towards self-antigens and manifested by the presence of circulating autoantibodies. The spectrum of autoimmune diseases comprises organ-specific forms with organ-specific antibodies (Hashimoto's thyroiditis, pernicious anaemia and thyrotoxicosis) and systemic diseases in which the antibodies are non-organ-specific (exemplified by systemic lupus erythematosus (SLE)). Intermediate types may be single organ disorders which are associated with autoantibodies that are not organ-specific. An example would be primary biliary cirrhosis in which there are circulating anti-smooth muscle and anti-mitochondrial antibodies.

There is a tendency for more than one type of single organ autoimmune disease to occur in the same individual, for example autoimmune thyroiditis occurring with pernicious anaemia. At the organ-specific end of the spectrum, immune destruction is mainly directed towards epithelial tissues derived from ectoderm or endoderm. The non-organ-specific autoimmune diseases centre upon tissues derived from mesoderm (e.g. blood, blood vessels, synovium and connective tissue). Autoimmune diseases are familial, age-related and occur more frequently in women than in men. Twin studies have indicated the importance of environmental factors such as infection as well as genetic constitution.

The example provided by tumour immunity makes it clear that tolerance as opposed to activation is the preferred option for the immune system. Autoimmunity is an exceptional state. An early concept in the study of single-organ autoimmunity was of sequestered antigens being released as a result of tissue injury. This still applies in the case of intra-ocular antigens, sperm and cardiac antigens, but does not explain the aetiology of the majority of cases. The underlying mechanisms are complex and ill understood, but are thought to involve the breakdown of cell regulation (activation of T helper cells; dysfunction of T suppressor cells) leading to the inappropriate stimulation of cytotoxic T cells and antibody producing B cells. Leaving aside the very real possibility that the antigen could in some cases be derived from as yet unidentified micro-organisms, the abnormal antigenic stimulation may be brought about by modification of autoantigens (e.g. by drugs), development of antibodies to micro-organisms that happen to cross-react with self-antigens (as in rheumatic heart disease in which antibodies against *Streptococcus pyogenes* react with the heart) and homologies between viruses and bacteria and T cell receptors.

Tissue destruction occurs through mechanisms comparable to those operating in type II (antibody-mediated cytotoxicity), type III (immune complex-mediated) or type IV (cell-mediated) hypersensitivity. Goodpasture's syndrome, in which the basement membrane of glomerular capillaries and pulmonary alveoli is attacked by complement fixing antibodies, is the classic example of type II hypersensitivity. In SLE, immune complexes are formed between antibodies and double-stranded DNA and are deposited in the kidneys and other organs. SLE is the most clear-cut example of autoimmune disease due to circulating immune complexes. As in hypersensitivity reactions, two or more of these mechanisms may apply to a single autoimmune disease. For example, T cells are likely to be implicated (at least in a regulatory capacity) in all forms of autoimmune disease, regardless of the participation of autoantibodies and immune complexes. However, direct invasion of tissues by B and T lymphocytes is seen in many single organ forms of autoimmune disease. It is likely that antibody- and cell-mediated cytodestruction occur in concert through antibody-dependent cell-mediated cytotoxicity (ADCC). The progressive endocrine failure of the thyroid gland in Hashimoto's disease and of the adrenal gland in Addison's disease results from organ atrophy. This in turn is caused by a relative increase in cell death over cell birth through activation of the apoptotic pathway (page 102).

REFERENCES

Scott, A.M. & Cebon, J. (1997) Clinical promise of tumour immunology. *Lancet,* **349** (Suppl II), 19–22.

Further reading

Chapel, H. & Haeney, M. (1993) *Essentials of Clinical Immunology* (3rd edn). Oxford: Blackwell Science.

Roitt, I. (1994) *Essential Immunology* (8th edn) . Oxford: Blackwell Scientific Publications.

— 31 —

ENVIRONMENTAL, IATROGENIC AND NUTRITIONAL DISEASE

The pathologist moves along step by step on solid ground;
the physiologist loops along, albeit part of the time in thin air

Fuller Albright

How may we recognise that a disorder is drug induced?

ENVIRONMENTAL FACTORS

Even if we are well nourished, grow and eat only our own vegetables, drink fresh spring water, avoid cigarettes, alcohol, hazardous occupations and leisure activities and all medications with side effects, and hide from the sun's ultraviolet light, we are still (leaving aside the microbiological agents waiting to strike at any moment) at risk from the environment. We cannot escape the environmental pollutants that we breathe, nor the ionising radiation (in the form of cosmic rays and radon gas derived from trace amounts of radioactive elements in the earth) that continuously bathes all living organisms (Pershagen et al., 1994).

Clearly, environmental factors impact on all disease processes, even those with a genetic basis. This chapter can provide only a cursory overview of this topic in keeping with the policy of classifying disease on the basis of disordered mechanisms operating at particular levels within the organism, and not according to the aetiological agent. Microbes, for example, are encompassed by the overarching category of inflammation. Similarly, the category of environmental agents covers inflammatory mechanisms (e.g. heat, cold, corrosive chemicals and physical trauma) (see Part II), vascular effects of diet (see Part III), and the carcinogenic effects of ultraviolet and ionising radiation, and other environmental mutagens (see Part IV).

IATROGENIC DISEASE

A major class of disease is iatrogenic disease caused by clinical management, particularly the administration of drugs with harmful side effects. Drug side effects are common, varied in their manifestations, and their consequences range from mild to life threatening.

204

Nevertheless, drugs remain in use because their benefits greatly outweigh their potential for harm. The possibility that particular signs or symptoms could be drug induced must always be considered and explored by taking a full drug history. The link may be obvious if, for example, a skin rash occurs soon after the administration of an antibiotic, whereas the connection may be less obvious if the patient is on many drugs, the side effects are internal, the complication has not been described previously, and/or the presentation is obscured by symptoms or signs of other disease. In such cases a very high level of suspicion will be required in order to reach the correct diagnosis.

Anatomical pathologists have made a considerable contribution to the initial recognition and description of the side effects of drugs that cause structural changes and affect internal organs such as the liver, gut, kidneys and lungs. The changes may be visible to the naked eye within surgically resected specimens, for example the ulcers and fibrous diaphragms that may form in the small intestine of subjects taking non-steroidal anti-inflammatory drugs (NSAIDS), or the neoplasms of the uterus or liver that may be associated with oestrogen. Lethal drug effects may be demonstrated at autopsy. These include venous thrombosis and pulmonary embolism caused by oestrogen, retroperitoneal fibrosis caused by beta blockers, pseudomembranous colitis caused by *Clostridium difficile* following the administration of broad spectrum antibiotics, or severe injury to the kidney (tubulointerstitial disease with papillary necrosis) caused by analgesics.

Because of its general role in drug metabolism and detoxification, the liver is a common site of drug-induced injury that will be manifested in both deranged liver function tests, and microscopically within liver biopsies. The type of injury and its anatomical distribution may point to the specific causative agent or at least to the underlying mechanism. The changes include fatty infiltration (tetracycline), cholestasis (steroids and chlorpromazine), granulomatous hepatitis, vasculitis and necrosis (halothane, paracetamol, isoniazid). The presence of eosinophils and granulomas points to a drug hypersensitivity.

Powerful drugs used in the treatment of cancer will likewise have powerful side effects. Anti-cancer drugs that act on dividing cells cause bone marrow suppression, pulmonary fibrosis (busulphan) and immunosuppression, and may initiate neoplasia. Immunosuppressive agents used to prevent organ rejection predispose the body to opportunistic infection by organisms such as cytomegalovirus, the protozoan Pneumocystis and fungi, and increase the risk of malignant lymphoma and multiple cutaneous tumours.

NUTRITIONAL DISEASE

Economic, social and psychological factors are the dominant causes of nutritional disease, but malnutrition can have an organic basis associated with diagnosable structural abnormalities. Both weight loss and iron deficiency anaemia may be due to malignancy. A cancer of the oesophagus may result in dysphagia, and patients with advanced cancer may be anorexic and subject to disordered metabolism causing the wasting known as cachexia. Diagnosis at this stage will be too late, but a bleeding cancer of the colon causing iron deficiency anaemia may be curable.

A variety of diseases of the intestinal tract may cause malabsorption manifested by loose fatty stools (steatorrhoea), weight loss and anaemia due to deficiency of iron and vitamins (principally B_{12} and folate). Intestinal biopsy will be especially helpful in the diagnosis of coeliac disease (gluten-sensitive enteropathy in which there is villous atrophy, crypt hyperplasia and intra-epithelial lymphocytosis), Crohn's disease, lymphoma and other rarer causes of malabsorption.

REFERENCES

Pershagen, G., Akerblom, G., Axelson, O., Clavensjo, B., Damber, L., Desai, G., Enflo, A., Lagarde, F., Mellander, H. & Svartengren, M., *et al.*(1994) Residential radon exposure and lung cancer in Sweden. *N Engl J Med,* **330**, 159–64.

Further reading

Warren, B.F. & Shepherd, N.A. (1995) Iatrogenic pathology of the gastrointestinal tract. In *Progress in Pathology*, volume 1, edited by N. Kirkham & P. Hall, pp. 31–54. Edinburgh: Churchill Livingstone.

32

MECHANICAL DISEASE

*I lived under a constant succession of fits of stone in the bladder,
till I was 26 years of age when the pain growing insupportable
I was delivered both of it and the stone by cutting*

Samuel Pepys (1633–1703)

What are the symptoms and signs of intestinal obstruction?

OBSTRUCTION

Although most of the disorders that afflict humankind involve complex mechanisms at the molecular level, one class of disease is relatively straightforward in the way in which it brings about its effects. Obstruction, which means the partial or complete blockage of the normal flow of solids, liquids or gases within any hollow tube or organ within the body, may be caused by simple mechanical events (the majority) or by more complex factors of a non-mechanical nature. The term obstruction without qualification is often used by surgeons to describe obstruction of the intestinal tract. Sudden obstruction to any large tube in the body is followed by serious and often life-threatening complications. The main sites of flow within the body include the gastrointestinal tract, the urinary tract, the cardiovascular system, the respiratory system, the genital tract and the ventricular system of the central nervous system.

Mechanical causes of obstruction can be divided into those in which the cause is found within the lumen of the hollow tube or organ, in the wall of the tube or organ or outside the wall.

Within the lumen

Obstruction of a lumen may be congenital (present at birth) due to a failure of development (atresia). Stones may form within a number of hollow organs including the gall bladder, the urinary tract and the ducts of salivary glands. Stones formed in the gall bladder may move from this site, causing colicky abdominal pain, and obstruct the common bile duct, causing jaundice. The passage of a stone within the urinary tract, particularly through the ureter, is associated with very severe and usually continuous pain radiating down the loin into the groin.

Abnormal secretions, notably the thick mucus associated with the inherited disorder cystic fibrosis (see below), may block bronchi in the lung and ducts in the pancreas. Five percent of infants with cystic fibrosis present soon after birth with intestinal obstruction due to an abnormal abundance of mucoid meconium (meconium ileus). Obstruction within the small intestine may be caused by the wall of the gut telescoping into the lumen (Fig. 39). Such an intussusception is usually provoked by a polypoid mass in the wall which is propelled forwards by peristaltic motion. The most common cause of obstruction within the cardiovascular system is thrombosis. This may cause obstruction where it is formed, or embolise within the circulation to impact elsewhere (see Chapter 18). A final cause of obstruction within the lumen is a foreign body.

Within the wall

A common cause of obstruction due to factors within the wall is a neoplasm, which may be benign or malignant. In the small intestine benign neoplasms or polyps usually cause obstruction by precipitating intussusception. Malignant neoplasms obstruct by producing a fibrous stricture. Strictures may also be caused by inflammatory processes such as peptic ulcers in the stomach and duodenum, Crohn's disease in the small and large intestine and diverticulitis in the sigmoid colon. The sphincter controlling the stomach outlet may be abnormally thickened in newborn infants, causing the condition pyloric stenosis. The abnormal fusion and thickening of heart valves may also be included in the category of intra-mural obstructing factors.

Outside the wall

Factors causing obstruction that are outside the wall are well described in the gut. The most common cause of small intestinal obstruction is a hernia (i.e. the abnormal protrusion of an organ through an anatomical boundary). Most hernias occur in the region of the groin (inguinal and femoral hernias) or the umbilicus. The gut may also become obstructed by fibrous bands or adhesions secondary to previous surgery or peritonitis. Redundant loops of bowel, for example the sigmoid colon, may twist around their pedicle, a condition known as volvulus. The latter is more common in people who eat very large amounts of vegetable fibre.

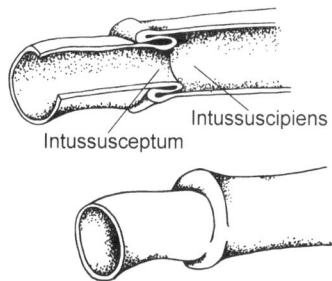

Figure 39 Small intestinal intussusception in which the 'intussusceptum' telescopes into the 'intussuscipiens'

Non-mechanical obstruction

Non-mechanical causes of obstruction in the gut relate to disorders of the plexus of nerves lying within the gut, or of the smooth muscle whose function it is to propel the contents forwards by peristaltic motion. In Hirschprung's disease ganglion cells are absent from the affected segment of bowel (usually the rectum), which then shows no peristaltic activity. This disease usually presents in the neonatal period or early childhood with severe constipation. Acquired damage to the nerve plexus may be caused by Chagas' disease (a parasitic disease of South America caused by the protozoan *Trypanosoma cruzi* which affects the oesophagus, other parts of the gut and the heart), by autoimmune destruction of the nerves or by degeneration of the smooth muscle (i.e. visceral myopathy). The most common cause of non-mechanical obstruction is paralytic ileus, in which the bowel ceases to function for several days following handling during abdominal surgery.

COMPLICATIONS OF OBSTRUCTION

Regardless of the cause or site of an obstruction, the effects are similar. Exaggerated peristaltic waves proximal to an obstructing lesion in intestine or ureter cause severe colicky pain. The pressure in the lumen ahead of or proximal to the obstruction will increase, causing dilatation. When the obstruction is longstanding, the smooth muscle in the wall will endeavour to force contents through the narrowed lumen and so undergo hypertrophy. Secretions will be retained within the obstructed organ and this stagnation will increase the likelihood of infection. Infection is a major complication of obstruction in the bronchial tree, biliary system and urinary tract. In the gut the build up of pressure may cause compression of intramural blood vessels leading to ischaemia and possibly necrosis of the wall. This may also lead to perforation which, (in the case of the gut), will cause peritonitis. Stones may form within stagnant secretions in longstanding obstruction of the urinary tract or salivary glands. Following obstruction within the pancreas or salivary glands the glands that normally release their products into the obstructed duct undergo shrinkage or atrophy.

When a loop of bowel becomes pinched off as in a hernia, or twisted as in torsion, the return of venous blood may be compromised and the tissues may become congested and oedematous, causing swelling. If the pressure built up compromises the arterial supply to the gut, the serious complications of ischaemic necrosis and gangrene will follow.

The male urethra passes through the prostate gland which commonly undergoes enlargement in later life. The resulting distortion to the urethra will impede the outflow of urine from the bladder, and the latter may undergo progressive enlargement as complete emptying fails. Urine may also reflux back into the ureters causing hydroureter and ultimately hydronephrosis, in which the pelvis of the kidney becomes greatly dilated. Complications of this will include renal failure, ascending infection and the formation of stones within the renal pelvis.

CYSTIC FIBROSIS

Simple obstruction of tubes in multiple organs by thick mucus is the basis of the severe complications of the inherited disorder cystic fibrosis. This autosomal recessive condition is one of the most common genetic diseases; about one in twenty five individuals is a carrier. Therefore 1 in 625 marriages is at risk, and 1 in 4 children of such a union is at risk of inheriting two mutated genes. The disease thereby affects about 1 in 2500, though is largely limited to Caucasians. The gene responsible for cystic fibrosis is on chromosome 7q31 and codes for a protein in the cell membrane that serves as a channel for the passage of chloride ions. The majority of mutations occur at the locus ΔF508.

Only about 5% of newborn infants with this condition develop meconium ileus, but this is life threatening without surgical intervention. In later life the most serious complications relate to the lungs and are due to plugging of the bronchi by mucus. Dilatation of the bronchi or bronchiectasis and severe lung infections follow. The mucus also blocks the ducts within the pancreas leading to loss of the glands that secrete digestive enzymes. The latter can be replaced artificially in the diet. Affected males are usually infertile because of obstruction of seminiferous tubules, and females may have anovulatory cycles as a consequence of chronic ill health.

33

END STAGE DISEASE

I know only that I do not know

Socrates

Why may it not be possible to achieve a definitive diagnosis?

INTRODUCTION

The term end stage disease describes the final stage in the natural evolution of a disease—the affected organ is then damaged beyond repair. Surprisingly the patient may be reasonably well, and sensitive laboratory tests of blood chemistry may show comparatively little abnormality. However, the end stage organ has lost its reserve function, and its capacity to maintain homeostasis (a stable internal environment) is limited. Only one small additional stimulus may be required to bring about organ failure and widespread metabolic disturbances. In order to survive, the patient will require either reversal of the precipitating event, artificial replacement of organ (e.g. renal dialysis) or an organ transplant.

End stage disease has other characteristics. It generally affects the entire organ in a diffuse way, though the mechanism underlying loss of function will vary within an organ as well as from one organ to another. The end point that is reached within a particular organ, however, may be similar regardless of the mode of injury. Without careful investigation it may be impossible to identify the underlying aetiology. Even with meticulous study, the cause of the end stage organ failure may remain a mystery. This is because tissues have a limited repertoire of responses to injury. When the tissue response develops over many years, progressive damage may obscure the earlier tissue changes that would have been diagnostic of a specific disease process. Coarse scarring, diffuse fibrosis, architectural disarray and atrophy may be all that is left. Epithelial tissues are replaced, surrounded or infiltrated by inert fibrous tissue in the anonymous end stage condition. Abnormal fibrosis is the common denominator in all end-stage disease.

END STAGE LIVER DISEASE

The ancient Greeks appeared, from the legend of Prometheus, to know that the liver has extraordinary powers of regeneration. According to this legend, Prometheus angered Zeus by handing over the gift of fire to mankind. As a punishment, Prometheus was chained to a rock and his liver eaten each day by a vulture, only to regenerate again. Normal liver will regenerate with full restoration of normal architecture when part of the organ is resected. However, regeneration will be imperfect when the connective tissue framework has been destroyed as a result of chronic injury, for example, in cirrhosis.

End stage liver disease, or cirrhosis, is characterised by diffuse involvement of the entire liver, nodular regeneration of hepatic parenchyma, fibrosis (which surrounds the nodules) and distortion of normal vascular relationships. Because the liver has multiple metabolic roles, cirrhotic patients present with numerous symptoms and signs, though these vary with the underlying cause of the process. Causes include viral infection (HBV and HCV), alcohol, biliary obstruction (primary and secondary), inherited disorders (haemochromatosis, α-1-antitrypsin deficiency, Wilson's disease, cystic fibrosis) and an idiopathic group in which autoimmunity plays a role. This list is not exhaustive but includes the most common causes. Medical history and serological tests for hepatitis virus or autoantibodies (anti-smooth muscle and anti-mitochondrial antibodies in the case of primary biliary cirrhosis) may point to a specific diagnosis in end stage disease. Additionally there may be diagnostic clues on both gross examination (surgery or autopsy) and microscopic examination (liver biopsy or autopsy) of the liver. In biliary cirrhosis (primary and secondary) the liver is often dark green because of cholestasis. Copper accumulates in the liver in Wilson's disease (an inherited disorder in which copper metabolism is impaired), and other liver diseases including primary biliary cirrhosis. In the latter, granulomas and lymphoid aggregates are typical histological findings. Excess iron deposition, particularly marked in the hepatocytes surrounding the portal tracts, characterises haemochromatosis. The brown pigment is obvious both macroscopically and microscopically and stains blue with Perls' stain. α-1-antitrypsin deficiency is associated with the presence of hepatocytes filled with PASd positive α-1-antitrypsin globules.

The nodules in cirrhosis following viral hepatitis tend to be large and associated with marked fibrosis. Special stains for HBV may be positive, notably by immunohistochemistry for HB antigens. By contrast, the nodules in alcoholic cirrhosis are small and associated with fine scarring. Active inflammation with neutrophil infiltration, Mallory's hyaline and fatty change (resulting in a pale liver macroscopically) may be seen in association with alcoholic cirrhosis. Despite the existence of these and other discriminators, a proportion of cases will defy a precise aetiological diagnosis.

END STAGE KIDNEY DISEASE

End stage kidney disease is characterised by the formation of shrunken, scarred kidneys, a relatively common autopsy finding. There are three principal sites for the injury that may precipitate renal failure: the blood supply, the glomeruli and the tubulo-interstitium.

Renal blood supply and ischaemic injury

The blood supply to the kidney may be compromised by two mechanisms that lead to shrinkage of the organ. First, atherosclerosis and arteriolosclerosis (see page 124) occur with increasing age but at an accelerated pace in subjects with longstanding hypertension.

Nephrons supplied by narrowed arterioles undergo atrophy and are replaced with scar tissue (nephrosclerosis). The intervening nephrons become hypertrophied to form raised 'granules' alternating with the scarred areas. The result is a finely granular contracted kidney. Second is atheroembolism and cholesterol crystal embolism originating mainly from atheromatous plaques in the descending aorta. Hypertension will again be a predisposing factor, together with the other risk factors for atherosclerosis (see Chapter 19). Multiple infarcts will result in coarse scarring. Because the kidney has considerable reserve capacity, nephrosclerosis on its own does not generally result in renal failure, but the combination of both mechanisms (hypertension and infarction) is not infrequent and may lead to renal impairment. This usually occurs in the elderly patient in whom there is an additional precipitating cause such as renal hypoperfusion due to septicemia or heart failure.

Glomeruli

Glomerulonephritis is an important cause of renal failure. This, however, is a general term describing many forms of glomerular injury with differing causes and outcomes. In end stage disease, the kidneys may be extremely small, be equal in size and show a fine surface granularity. Glomerular sclerosis is not caused by the accumulation of type I collagen that occurs with the usual scarring of chronic inflammation, but rather by basement membrane material (type IV collagen and laminin) and matrix derived from the mesangium (the interstitium of the glomerulus containing mesangial cells). Because patients with glomerulonephritis develop hypertension, the changes of nephrosclerosis may be superimposed upon those of glomerulonephritis.

Tubules and interstitium

In tubulointerstitial disease, the focus of inflammation is upon the interstitial connective tissue and the renal tubules. There are multiple causes, including repeated bacterial infection, obstruction of renal outflow and analgesic abuse (e.g. phenacetin) with associated papillary necrosis. Grossly the kidneys are shrunken with coarse scars, and often appear asymmetrical. An infective cause may be suspected from the patient's history, through examination of the gross specimen for evidence of active inflammation in the collecting system and by the presence of lymphoid aggregates on histology. However, the histological appearance of 'thyroidisation' (dilated tubules filled with pink homogenous material resembling colloid) may also be formed in ischaemic kidneys. Additionally, ischaemic and hypertensive changes may be superimposed leading to secondary nephrosclerosis.

In diabetic end stage renal disease, all three anatomical sites may be implicated: arterioles (efferent as well as afferent), glomeruli and tubulo-interstitium. The preceding examples illustrate how multiple disease processes within three principal anatomical sites of activity may ultimately converge to give an overlapping morphology. Nevertheless, even in the end stages subtle clues may allow the list of possible underlying diagnoses to be at least narrowed down.

END STAGE LUNG DISEASE

As with the kidney, multiple types of injury centred on different anatomical structures may drive the lung towards slowly progressive failure that is irreversible. The disease processes include emphysema, bronchiectasis, cryptogenic fibrosing alveolitis, lung fibrosis due to industrial dust exposure (pneumoconiosis), and pulmonary hypertension. However the morphological change (not disease) that best lends itself to the concept of end stage lung disease comparable with cirrhosis is 'honeycomb lung'. This results from the destruction of alveolar tissue, forming large air spaces bounded by fibrous tissue with total destruction of normal architecture in the affected areas. Less affected lung must exist elsewhere, otherwise gas exchange could not have sustained life. Honeycombing occurs in some of the above named conditions, specifically those in which there is extensive interstitial fibrosis—cryptogenic fibrosing alveolitis, asbestosis, berylliosis, sarcoidosis (an idiopathic condition associated with granulomatous inflammation)—and in some subjects who recover from adult respiratory distress syndrome.

CONCLUSION

Patients with end stage disease affecting the liver, kidney or lung may have been treated for many years following a definitive diagnosis of a specific disorder known to follow a chronic and progressive course. Alternatively, symptoms may have presented at a relatively late stage in the natural history of the condition. The patient is often relatively young. If the patient is elderly or frail, autopsy examination may provide the only opportunity to investigate the underlying cause. Although widespread fibrosis, loss of functioning parenchyma and architectural distortion are common to all forms of end stage disease, residual diagnostic clues may point to a specific aetiology. It is generally desirable to reach a definitive diagnosis even if this is reached too late to help the patient. The incidence of a disease, its changing frequency over time and the frequent involvement of environmental factors in the causation of end stage disease are all very real public health concerns. The possibility of industrial exposure to harmful dusts or fibres may have legal implications in terms of compensation for the individual's family. In short, organ failure is not a diagnosis.

FURTHER READING

Gibbs, A.R. & Seal, R.M.E. (1982) *Atlas of Pulmonary Pathology*. Lancaster: MTP Press.
Heptinstall, R.H. (1992) End-stage renal disease. In *Pathology of the Kidney* (4th edn), edited by R.H. Heptinstall, pp. 713–777. Boston: Little, Brown and Co.
Kincaid-Smith, P. & Becker, G. (1978) Reflux nephropathy and chronic atrophic pyelonephritis: a review. *J Infect Dis,* **138**, 589–93.

Resolve to be always beginning—to be a beginner

Rainer Maria Rilke

GLOSSARY

Abscess. A collection of pus

Adenocarcinoma. A cancer (malignant neoplasm) derived from glandular tissues.

Adenoma. A benign neoplasm (tumour) composed of glandular tissue.

Adhesion molecules. A large family of molecules occurring at the surfaces of cells; they allow cells to adhere to other cells of the same or different type, or to connective tissue elements such as collagen.

Adipocyte. A fat cell.

Aetiology. The primary cause of a disease.

Alkaptonuria. An autosomal recessive disorder caused by a failure to metabolise homogentisic acid. This accumulates in tissues (cartilage) which become black (ochronosis).

Allele. One of a pair of hereditary units (genes).

Amyloidosis. Deposition of an eosinophilic, Congo red positive proteinaceous material between cells in various tissues of the body and in a variety of clinical settings.

Aneurysm. A focal dilatation within the cardiovascular system which may rupture spontaneously causing catastrophic haemorrhage.

Angiogenesis. The process of developing new blood vessels (neovascularisation)

Antibody. A molecule produced by B-lymphocytes (plasma cells) which serves to opsonise bacteria (prepare them for phagocytosis) and neutralise viruses and toxins. Known also as an immunoglobulin, the protein includes a specific sequence of amino acids allowing it to interact only with the antigen that provoked its production.

Antigen. Any substance capable of producing an immune response, such as the production of an antibody.

APC. 1. A tumour suppressor gene named after the inherited condition adenomatous polyposis coli (see FAP), and the first commonly occurring tumour suppressor gene to be identified through the study of a rare familial type of cancer. 2. Antigen presenting cell.

Atheroma. Localised intimal thickening associated with fibrosis, accumulation of lipid and smooth muscle cell proliferation.

Atherosclerosis. The process of arterial injury ('hardening') that is caused by inflammatory damage affecting the intimal lining of the vessel.

ATP. Adenosine triphosphate, a high energy form of the nucleoside adenosine.

Atrophy. Acquired reduction in the size of a cell or organ.

Autopsy. The postmortem examination of a body, the term meaning literally to see for oneself. Also described as necropsy.

Autosome. A chromosome other than an X or Y chromosome.

215

Basal cell carcinoma. A common type of (non-metastasising) skin cancer.

Base. In the context of DNA and RNA, this term describes the chemical compounds adenine and guanine (purines), and thymine, cytosine and uracil (pyrimidines). Linked to a simple sugar (deoxyribose) molecule, the bases are termed nucleosides (adenosine, guanosine, thymidine, cytidine and uridine). Within DNA or RNA, the nucleosides are phosphorylated as nucleotides.

Biopsy. The removal and examination of a small piece of tissue in order to achieve a diagnosis by microscopic investigation.

Calcification. The laying down of calcium in tissues. Dystrophic calcification occurs in diseased tissues and metastatic calcification occurs in normal tissues as a result of hypercalcemia (raised plasma calcium).

Carbohydrate. A class of molecules including simple sugars, starches, plant fibers and gums.

Carcinogenesis. Mechanism underlying evolution of cancer.

Carcinoid. Neoplasm derived from cells of the diffuse endocrine system.

Carcinoma. Malignant neoplasm of epithelial origin.

Carcinoma in situ. Carcinoma that is still limited to an epithelial surface (i.e. has not invaded through the basement membrane or developed the potential to spread to distant sites).

CD. Cluster designation. Agreed nomenclature for leukocyte cell membrane antigens.

Chemical pathology. The branch of laboratory medicine involved with the detection and quantification of chemical substances in blood, urine and other fluids.

Chemotaxin. Chemical attractant of motile cells.

Chemotherapy. Treatment (generally of cancer) with chemical agents.

Chromatin. Material within the nucleus of the cell made up of DNA and protein.

Chromosome. A discrete unit within the nucleus of the cell comprising multiple genes. A human cell contains twenty-two pairs of chromosomes together with either two X chromosomes (in females) or an X and a Y chromosome (in males).

Cirrhosis. A disease of the liver in which the normal architecture is permanently altered and liver function is impaired. Alcohol and hepatitis viruses are important causes but there are also many others.

Clone. To reproduce multiple copies of a cell (or gene) from a single cell (or gene). Cloning of a gene implies that the gene has been localised within a particular chromosome, isolated and sequenced (meaning that the sequence of bases has been determined).

Coagulation. The process of clotting culminating in the conversion of fibrinogen to fibrin.

Coagulative necrosis. The most common type of ischaemic necrosis.

Codon. The sequence of three bases in DNA which codes for a specific amino acid (the building blocks of proteins).

Collagen. A protein found in the extracellular matrix of connective tissues which is either fibrillary or amorphous in structure.

Complement. The system of plasma enzymes which facilitates the acute inflammatory process.

Congenital. Present at birth.

Congestion. The accumulation of blood within an organ due to reduced venous outflow.

Connective tissue. Tissue that supports and provides the structural framework for parenchymal tissues. The key connective tissue cell is the collagen secreting fibroblast.

Crohn's disease. Chronic granulomatous inflammatory disorder affecting the gut (mainly the intestines).

Cyst. A collection of fluid or semi-solid material within a sac with an epithelial lining.

Cytokine. A chemical mediator or growth factor secreted by cells (principally lymphocytes and monocyte-derived cells).

Cytopathology. A laboratory diagnostic service involving the microscopic study of cells as opposed to tissues (e.g. cervical smears).

Desmoplasia. The formation within a cancer of a dense collagenous stroma.

Differentiation. The process whereby specialised cells are derived from uncommitted stem cells (see stem cells).

Diverticulum. A blind ending sac.

DNA. Deoxyribonucleic acid, which constitutes the primary genetic material of most living organisms and is composed of four bases (G, C, A and T) (see base). DNA is duplicated by replication and forms the template for transcribing RNA (see RNA).

DNA repair gene. A gene which normally repairs genetic damage but fails to do so when it is itself mutated or lost. Mutation or loss of both copies leads to a state of hypermutability and hence carcinogenesis.

Dominant. Describes a hereditary effect caused by a single mutated gene.

Dysplasia. Disordered growth and differentiation. Sometimes used to indicate a pre-invasive neoplastic change (e.g. in the gut).

Ectasia. Dilatation of a duct or tube.

Effusion. An exudate in a serous cavity (pericardial, pleural or peritoneal).

Electron microscope. A microscope employing a beam of electrons instead of a light source in order to achieve magnification beyond the range of a light microscope ($\leftrightarrow$1,000 to $\leftrightarrow$500,000).

Embolism. The passage of a mass within the bloodstream from a point of origin to a point of impaction.

Endoplasmic reticulum. The cytoplasmic system of membranous cisternae which is the site of protein synthesis (rough) and lipid synthesis (smooth).

Endothelial cell. A flattened and highly versatile cell lining blood vessels and forming the endothelium.

Enzyme. A biological molecule, usually a protein, which catalyses (activates) chemical reactions.

Eosinophil. A white blood cell with large eosinophilic granules with multiple inflammatory roles.

Epithelium. Tissue which lines hollow organs or covers surfaces such as the skin.

Exudate. Inflammatory outpouring of fluid derived from plasma into an extracellular site. It may be serous (protein rich and straw coloured), serosanguinous (protein rich and blood-stained), fibrinous (comprising abundant fibrin) or purulent (cream coloured due to presence of pus cells).

Familial. Describes a condition that is inherited and therefore affects multiple family members.

Familial adenomatous polyposis (FAP). An inherited disorder caused by mutation of the APC gene in which affected subjects develop multiple precancerous polyps (adenomas) of the large intestine.

Fat necrosis. A form of necrosis complicating acute pancreatitis that is accompanied by calcification. May also be caused by trauma, for example to breast.

Fibrin. The coagulated form of the plasma protein fibrinogen.

Fibrinoid necrosis. Describes an appearance seen in vasculitis (acute inflammation of vessel wall) in which there is fibrin deposition. A misnomer since necrosis may not be demonstrable.

Fibroblast. A spindle shaped connective tissue cell which secretes collagen.

Fibrosis. The laying down of collagen-rich connective tissue.

Fine needle aspiration. A form of biopsy in which groups of cells are obtained by means of a fine needle.

Fistula. A track connecting two epithelial surfaces that is lined by granulation tissue.

Gangrene. A combination of necrosis (usually ischaemic) and bacterial invasion causing putrefaction.

Gene. A sequence of DNA coding for a single protein.

Germ cell. A cell responsible for the generation of sperm or ova.

Glycogen. A large molecule formed of glucose, and the form in which glucose is stored.

Grade. In relation to cancer describes the level of aggressiveness (low grade = low aggressiveness, high grade = high aggressiveness).

Granulation tissue. A newly generated form of connective tissue involved in the process of healing.

Granuloma. A localised collection of macrophages (histiocytes).

Granulomatous inflammation. A form of chronic inflammation in which granulomas are present.

Haematology. The branch of laboratory and clinical medicine focusing on diseases of the blood (leukaemia, anaemia and bleeding disorders).

Haemosiderin. The form in which iron is stored. A partially denatured form of ferritin.

Haemostasis. The physiological process of haemorrhage arrest.

Heat shock proteins. A family of proteins which rescue other proteins following cell injury.

Helicobacter pylori. A bacterium responsible for chronic inflammation of the lining of the stomach (chronic gastritis).

Hereditary non-polyposis colorectal cancer (HNPCC). An inherited form of large intestinal cancer caused by mutation in a DNA mismatch repair gene.

Hilum. Indented or central point of an organ at which vessels, ducts or nerves enter and leave.

Histamine. An inflammatory mediator stored in mast cell, platelets and other tissues, which causes vasodilatation and increased vascular permeability.

Histogenetic. A form of classification of neoplasms (tumours) based on the tissue type constituting the lesion.

Histopathology. The branch of laboratory medicine that is equivalent to anatomical pathology or surgical pathology.

Hormone. A chemical messenger (usually a protein or steroid) produced by an endocrine gland. Following its release into the blood stream a hormone acts on tissues at a distant site.

Humour. One of four fluids believed (from the time of the ancient Greeks until the nineteenth century) to underlie states of health and disease. An excess of one of these (black bile) was thought to be the cause of cancer.

Hyaline. Microscopic appearance that is pink, homogeneous and 'glassy'.

Hydropic swelling. A form of reversible cell injury.

Hyperaemia. Increased volume of blood in an organ caused by increased arterial flow.

Hyperplasia. An increase in cell numbers leading to enlargement of a tissue or organ.

Hypersensitivity. Excessive and destructive immune response.

Hypertrophy. An increase in the size of a cell or organ.

Hypoxia. A state of reduced supply of oxygen.

Immunoglobulin. A type of protein which functions as an antibody. There are five classes: IgG, IgM, IgA, IgD and IgE.

Immunohistochemistry. A form of tissue staining utilising the specific binding properties of antibodies.

Infarct. An area of ischaemic necrosis. Infarction is the process of ischaemic necrosis.

Ischaemia. Reduction of blood supply to tissues.

Karyolysis. Dissolution of nuclei seen in a necrotic cell.

Karyorrhexis. Fragmentation of nuclei seen in a necrotic cell.

Kupffer cell. A macrophage found in the liver.

Labile. A cell type which proliferates continuously.

Leukaemia. Malignancy of white blood cells—lymphocytes, monocytes or myeloid cells.

Linkage. The close proximity of two genetic sites (loci) within a chromosome.

Lipofuscin. A brown wear-and-tear pigment found in autophagic vacuoles.

Liquefactive necrosis. A type of ischaemic necrosis in which tissues liquefy. Cerebral infarction is notable for being followed by liquefactive necrosis.

Lymphatic system. A system of fine vessels which serves to conduct excess fluid from the spaces surrounding cells (interstitium) back into the blood system. See lymph nodes.

Lymph node. A bean-sized organ ('gland') found throughout the lymphatic system conmprising lymphocytes and other cells responsible for immune defense.

Lymphocyte. A white blood cell responsible for the orchestration of immunity to infection by micro-organisms. B lymphocytes produce antibodies, and T lymphocytes have helper (CD4), suppressor (CD8) and cytotoxic (CD8) roles.

Lymphoma. A malignant tumour of lymphoid cells arising in lymph nodes or extranodal sites where lymphocytes aggregate together.

Lysosomes. Cytoplasmic organelles containing enzymes used in autophagy and phagocytosis.

Lysozyme. An enzyme which lyses bacterial cell walls. Also known as muramidase.

Macrophage. A large phagocytic cell with multiple inflammatory functions.

Malignant. An adjective indicating the cancerous nature of a lesion (having the capacity for local invasion and metastasis).

Malignant melanoma. A malignant tumour composed of melanin-producing cells (melanocytes) arising in the skin and rarely in other sites.

Mast cell. A cell found in connective tissues containing inflammatory mediators (such as histamine) in basophilic granules.

Meiosis. A form of cell division leading to the generation of gametes (sperm or ova).

Melanin. Dark brown pigment produced by melanocytes of skin. The cytoplasmic organelles secreting melanin are called melanosomes.

Meningioma. A benign central nervous tissue tumour (usually) which is derived from meningeal coverings of the brain.

Mesenchyme. Undifferentiated tissue of mesodermal origin which gives rise to connective tissue including such specialised tissues as bone, cartilage, muscle and vessels.

Metaplasia. Change in the direction of differentiation by a tissue.

Metastasis. The process of spread of malignant cells to form colonies in distant sites (secondary deposits of cancer).

Microbiology. The branch of laboratory medicine involved with the identification of infective micro-organisms and the management of infection.

Microsatellites. Non-coding regions in the genome composed of repeating sequences of bases and showing marked variation between individuals.

Mitochondria. Cytoplasmic organelles that are the seat of aerobic respiration.

Mitosis. Division of a cell into two identical daughter cells.

Monoclonal antibody. An antibody produced by a clone of antibody-producing cells.

Monocyte. A circulating white blood cell which becomes a macrophage when it leaves the bloodstream.

Mucin. Viscid material composed of glycoprotein that is secreted by some glandular epithelia.

Mutagen. Agent causing genetic mutation.

Mutation. Alteration in the structure of a gene.

Natural killer (NK) cell. A killing lymphocyte that is neither a B cell nor a T cell (null cell).

Necrosis. Morphological change following cell death. May be coagulative, liquefactive, caseous or fat necrosis.

Neoplasm. A new growth which may be either benign or malignant. A malignant neoplasm is a cancer.

Neutrophil. A white blood cell also known as a polymorphonuclear leukocyte which phago-cytoses bacteria. The main cell type involved in acute inflammation.

Nosology. The systematic classification of disease.

Nucleolus. A nuclear body that is the site of ribosomal RNA synthesis.

Oedema. Presence of increased amounts of fluid within the extracellular compartment.

Oligodendroglioma. A malignant tumour of the central nervous system derived from the oligodendrocyte (a myelin-secreting cell).

Oncogene. A cancer gene that is an activated or mutated form of a proto-oncogene.

Oncology. The study or clinical management of cancer.

Organisation. Removal of dead tissue, fibrin or thrombus and its replacement by connective tissue.

Parenchyma. The cellular or functional elements of an organ that fill the connective tissue framework or stroma.

Pathogenesis. The mechanism of evolution of a disease.

Permanent. Describes cells with no capacity for division.

Pernicious anemia. An autoimmune disease in which antibodies are directed towards the parietal cells of the stomach. Parietal cells secrete acid and intrinsic factor (necessary for absorption of vitamin B_{12}). B_{12} deficiency causes dysmaturation of red blood cells which become enlarged (megaloblastic).

Phagocytosis. The engulfment and digestion of foreign particles or cellular debris by white blood cells (neutrophils or macrophages).

Phase contrast. A form of light microscopy which is useful for studying whole cells and living cells.

Plasma cell. A cell derived from the B lymphocyte which produces antibodies.

Platelet. A cytoplasmic fragment derived from megakaryocytes and involved in coagulation (thrombotic aggregation) and inflammation.

Polyp. A descriptive term meaning a small, mushroom-like growth arising from an epithelial surface.

Precancerous lesion. A histological change (sometimes described as dysplasia) associated with an increased risk of malignant transformation.

Prognosis. The predicted outlook for a patient with a serious disease such as cancer.

Protein. A fundamental molecule in all life-forms, built of amino acids and encoded in DNA. Proteins function as enzymes, hormones, receptors and various structural filaments within cells.

Proto-oncogene. A gene implicated in normal cellular division which, when mutated, becomes an oncogene.

Psammoma body. A microscopic calcified body found in several types of neoplasm.

Pus. Thick yellow material formed of dead and dying neutrophils.

Pyknosis. Shrinkage and increased staining intensity of nuclei seen in damaged and/or necrotic cells.

Radiology. The demonstration of internal anatomy by means of X-rays and other imaging modalities.

Radiotherapy. The treatment of disease (cancer) by means of ionising radiation.

Reagent. A chemical agent which reacts with another agent (substrate) to yield a product.

Recessive. Describes an inherited effect observed when both copies of a gene (both alleles) are mutated.

Regeneration. Restoration of normal structure and function.

Reperfusion injury. Damage to reperfused ischaemic tissue caused by the formation of active oxygen species.

Restriction fragment length polymorphism. Variation in the structure of DNA from person to person that is demonstrated by the cutting of DNA into fragments of differing length by means of restriction enzymes.

Retinoblastoma. A tumour of childhood arising in the retina of the eye.

Ribosome. A form of RNA from which protein synthesis occurs (translation). Ribosomes are attached to endoplasmic reticulum (rough).

RNA. Ribonucleic acid. This nucleic acid is transcribed from DNA and forms the template for the translation of a protein product.

Sarcoidosis. A disorder of unknown aetiology in which non-caseating granulomatous inflammation occurs in multiple tissues and organs.

Sarcoma. A malignant neoplasm arising from connective tissue.

Screening. A population-based exercise that seeks to prevent disease or detect it at an early and curative stage, thereby reducing the incidence of disease-related death or morbidity within the screened community.

Sex-linked. Describes a gene that is linked to (i.e. resides on) a chromosome that determines gender (X chromosome in practice). In sex-linked recessive conditions, males are affected and females are carriers (usually).

Shock. A state of cardiovascular collapse resulting in generalised tissue hypoperfusion and hypotension when compensatory mechanisms fail.

Sinus. A blind ending track opening onto an epithelial surface and lined by granulation tissue.

Somatic. Relating to cells of the body apart from germ cells.

Squamous cell carcinoma. A common form of cancer arising from the skin, cervix or lung.

Stable. Describes cells which are capable of division when provoked but which show little mitotic activity under normal circumstances.

Stage. A system indicating the extent of spread of a cancer.

Stem cell. An immortal and uncommitted cell capable of differentiating into multiple cell types.

Substrate. A chemical compound (for example produced by a cell) that yields a product when acted upon by a reagent.

Telomerase. An enzyme which reconstitutes telomeres.

Telomere. The terminal portion of chromosome involved in chromosomal stability which shortens with each cell division. Implicated in ageing and cancer.

Thromboembolism. An embolism made of thrombus.

Thrombosis. Aggregation of platelets into a mass accompanied by deposition of fibrin.

Thymus. The lymphoid organ in which T lymphocytes are generated.

Tissue. An aggregation of cells of one type into an organised whole.

Toxin. A chemical which causes cell injury. A more specific microbiological meaning is a bacterial product which provokes injury that is accompanied by an inflammatory or immunological response. The product may be soluble (exotoxin) or associated with the bacterial cell wall (endotoxin).

Transcription. Generation of messenger RNA from the DNA template.

Translation. Generation of protein from the RNA template.

Transudate. Protein-poor fluid collection within an extracellular site that is derived from the circulating blood.

Tumour. This word literally means swelling but is used to indicate a neoplasm, either benign or malignant.

Tumour suppressor gene. A variety of cancer gene that subserves different normal functions. When both copies are mutated or lost, the cessation of the normal function provokes malignant behaviour of the cell.

Ulcer. Localised loss of an epithelial lining or surface.

Ulcerative colitis. A chronic (long-standing) disease of the large intestine associated with inflammation and ulceration.

Vasculitis. Inflammation of vessels.

Virus. The smallest infective agent that is an obligate parasite (requires the genetic machinery of a host cell to complete its life cycle). Genetic material of a virus may be either DNA or RNA. Individual viral particles can be seen through an electron microscope but not through a light microscope.

Wild type. The functioning (non-mutated) form of a gene.

INDEX

Page numbers in italics indicate a definition in the glossary.